EVERYTHING
UNDER
THE SUN

EVERYTHING UNDER THE SUN

A FAMILY DOCTOR'S REFLECTIONS ON LIFE, LOVE, LOSS AND RENEWED HOPE IN MEDICINE

BRUCE ROWE, MD

Everything Under the Sun: A Family Doctor's Reflections
On Life, Love, Loss and Renewed Hope in Medicine

For information about this title or to order other books and/
or electronic media, contact the publisher:

Bruce E. Rowe, MD
Brown Deer, Wisconsin
browehawkeye@gmail.com
https://bowtiedocblog.com

ISBNs:
978-1-7340202-0-5 (softcover)
978-1-7340202-1-2 (eBook)

Printed in the United States of America

Cover and Interior design: 1106 Design

Disclaimer

Wherever appropriate, patient vignettes were utilized with the expressed permission of the persons involved. Out of appreciation and respect for their privacy, their names and identifying details have been changed. With the passage of time, precise recollection of life events often blur and fade, and reasonable people could disagree on what exactly occurred with respect to a specific incident. I have attempted to reconstruct and share my life narrative to the best of my ability, with an accurate retelling of my personal experiences as I currently perceive them. My goal is to be entertaining and informative, but most importantly, truthful and not present situations in an inflated positive or artificially negative light.

For Laura, Allison, Chelsea and Julia,
beloved companions on my life's greatest journey

TABLE OF CONTENTS

FOREWORD

Medicine is Changing. Ever since I set foot in the door for my medical school orientation in the fall of 1990, I have heard that phrase uttered countless times by supervising physicians, fellow residents and aspiring medical students. The context for the comment was almost universally negative; somehow that the profession of being a physician had lost its luster and joyfulness, never to be retrieved again. Many of my fellow doctors have looked back on the previous eras of medicine with a sense of resigned wistfulness in that we arrived to the party too late. Modern-day physicians face less prestige and more scrutiny and regulation on a regular basis. Administrative tasks such as obtaining insurance authorization, completing paperwork, and navigating complicated electronic medical records (EMRs) have intruded upon the physician-patient relationship in increasingly extensive and sinister ways. The joyfulness and special nature of the doctor's visit is under siege unlike any other time in the history of medical practice.

These concerning changes have been felt not only on a systemic level in health-care delivery, but also within the individual personality of each personal physician. Depression, burnout and depersonalization have reached epidemic levels in the medical practitioner community. Suicide claims the life of a physician at the rate of one per day, an astronomical figure. Each year, 360+ doctors leave a spouse, children and their patients without the love, support and healing that they need and deserve.

The inspiration to write this book emanated from two primary issues. First, I became alarmed at how the modern constraints of medicine were adversely affecting the health care system and potentially my patients. Second, like many of my fellow physicians, I began to experience feelings of sadness, burnout and being overwhelmed by the demands of my medical practice. Dreading the busy clinic days, becoming frustrated with patients and feeling helpless to make things better in my community contributed to a sense that I was "losing my edge," so to speak. I hated how I felt and worried about my negative energy impacting my patients.

After many hours of meditation, prayer and reflection, I decided to place my thoughts and life experiences on paper not only for my own healing, but also to guide others who are undergoing periods of discouragement and loss of confidence. I needed to reestablish the self-affirmation that I made the right decision in dedicating my life to serving as a family physician, while maintaining a faith that we all can affect positive changes within our respective health-care networks.

So to my fellow physicians, I exhort: *Keep showing up and giving your absolute best every single day.* It is critical for all

health-care professionals to know that what they do for their
families, communities and patients *matters,* and that the world
is a better place because of their sacrifice and commitment to the
health and happiness of the human soul. This memoir with my
life journey displayed through its multiple vignettes is dedicated
in part to those who work hard to maintain the health of their
fellow man, woman and child every day.

—BRUCE ROWE, MD
September 2019

CHAPTER 1

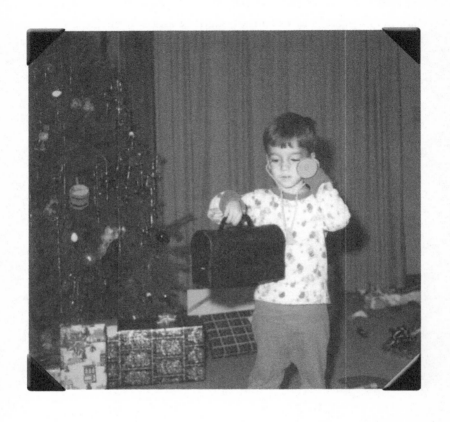

MORNING

Daybreak made a dramatic entrance, with a sliver of brightness bursting through a gap in my bedroom window shade, followed by an unceremonious beeping of my alarm clock. I have never been much of a morning person, but I needed to awaken and prepare for work. The majestic sun ascended, an orange ball illuminating my suburban Milwaukee home nestled along the western shores of Lake Michigan. Steadily I roused myself and struggled to mobilize in bed, like an aspiring seedling emerging from the fertile loam of my native Iowa farm fields. I reluctantly turned onto my right side and glanced at the digit readout on my bedside clock radio. *6:15 a.m. . . . on a Monday!*

Man . . . is it really morning already?

"You'd better get a move on, Doc, you have a busy day ahead and you don't want to get behind early!" my wife called out in an all-too enthusiastic voice from downstairs. She dubbed me "Doc" long before I became a practicing family physician, and I love it. I finally extricated myself from the seducing comfort of my pillow and began to mentally prepare for the fast-approaching morning of rounds and clinic. As I hustled out the door, I gave her a brief yet heartfelt smooch as I embarked on another adventurous day.

I hope that I am ready to take on today, I contemplated cautiously as I arrived at my clinic. It was 8:45 a.m., a day already filled with interesting patient moments. On morning hospital rounds, I met Drew, a healthy newborn baby; checked in on Frank, a gregarious Italian gentleman with heart failure; my nursing home lady Edna with pneumonia and sepsis, concluding with Florence, a beautiful eighty-year-old woman on the hospice unit gracefully braving the terminal phases of metastatic colon cancer. We lovingly clasped our hands together and cried, reflecting upon a beautiful life that would soon come to an end—*it had been one helluva run.*

Settling into my office chair, I reviewed the day's schedule, attempting to anticipate each patient's potential issues and treatment plans. The list of appointments was a rich tapestry of people and problems which defined the family physician's medical practice: young and old, routine and urgent visits, healthy and seriously ill. Walk-in patients would make unexpected appearances, often with deceptive medical concerns which could be amazingly easy or devastatingly complicated. The innumerable curious medical elements hiding daily behind these exam room doors attracted me to the nebulous and unpredictable world of the family doctor.

I was immersed in the demands of the daily schedule, answering messages, reviewing patient lab results and answering email, when my medical assistant Latisha came into my office and caught my attention.

"Maddie's ready for you . . . she hurt her elbow this morning, she and her mother are really upset."

Maddie was a sweet, nearly three-year-old girl whom I have cared for since she was a newborn baby. Her normally happy and loving mother appeared to be stricken with a sense of guilt and sadness.

"Hi Maddie, it's Dr. Bruce here," I began pleasantly, conveying reassurance. "What happened to your elbow?"

"My elbow hurts, I no move it," she said tearfully and with a slight measure of defiance. I looked over at mom, who was blinking furiously in a hopeful effort to overcome her moist eyes. She gathered herself and recounted the unfortunate event:

"I was trying to get Maddie ready for daycare, but she pulled away from me when I was trying to get her jammies off. Then she said her right elbow hurt, and she stopped moving it. I really hope I didn't break her arm . . . I feel so bad about what happened."

I smiled warmly at Maddie and mom with comfort and understanding. "I don't think anything is broken. It could be a nursemaid's elbow, which we should be able to fix."

Nursemaid's elbow, or radial head subluxation, is a condition when a structure called the annular ligament slips off the head of the radius bone in the elbow, usually due to a toddler pulling away from a parent. This strong traction and parent-child tug-of-war often results in the ligament being displaced and the child being reluctant to move the arm at all. At this point, the parents often fear the worst; but the ligament misplacement can simply be corrected by extending the elbow and arm, rotating the hand out and away from the body and placing a thumb with gentle, steady pressure over the radial head. The maneuver is performed over a few brief seconds, and usually if the radial head is restored to its proper position, the doctor will sense a distinctive click or slight pop.

After getting her mother's approval, I turned my attention to Maddie, who was apprehensive, unusually reserved and had her arm strongly attached to the side of her chest, elbow tightly flexed, stubbornly resisting all arm movement. Gently, I coaxed her to let me look at her elbow, and as I deftly performed the reduction maneuver, I encountered the anticipated wonderful, satisfying click. She gave a slight gasp, but within two to three minutes she was moving her right arm and elbow once again in a normal fashion.

Maddie's mom was ecstatic. "Oh, I'm so relieved! I'm glad it wasn't broken. Thanks, Dr. Rowe! Does she need a sling or anything?"

"Nope," I replied proudly. "She should be just fine now. Try not to pull on her arm or elbow area, especially if she's resisting you."

Feeling relieved and accomplished, I happily moved on to the next patient. It was already a bustling morning, with my exam rooms filling, discharging and replacing patients in a repetitive cycle. Esther was a seventy-eight-year-old Jewish widow who still played golf and mah-jongg twice per week. She was petite, with a beautiful smile, healthy olive skin, and her gray-streaked black hair was always immaculately done. She was here for a recheck of her hypertension, diabetes and high cholesterol issues. A review of her labs from last week showed excellent results and control. I congratulated Esther on her efforts and good report, and for the remainder of the visit we mixed medical discussions with updates on her grandchildren and her putting game. The interaction was enjoyable and mutually therapeutic. As we finished our visit, she said, "Thanks for taking such good care of me, Dr. Rowe. I'm so lucky to have you as my physician."

"You're welcome, Esther . . . remember, long and straight down the fairway!" She smiled pleasantly, and as she turned to depart, burst forth with a sweet, heartfelt laugh.

Jessica was a twenty-six-year-old single mother of two young children under the age of five, with a long-standing history of depression. Adding insult to injury, she had recently lost her job. After confirming that she had no active thoughts of harming or killing herself, I spent some extra time giving her encouragement and suggesting various coping techniques. I restarted her antidepressant medication and referred her back to a counselor for further psychotherapy. We both knew that Jessica had a significant journey in front of her, but after our appointment, both of us believed that ultimate success was possible.

Jessica gathered herself to leave, gave me a tear-soaked hug, and after she deployed a honk-like nasal clearing into a Kleenex, said, "Thanks, Dr. Rowe, I feel better already after just talking with you. Hopefully the counselor can help me out too."

"And please call me in one week to give me an update," I gently reminded her. Depressed people need a sense of restored hopefulness and connectivity with others. As we strolled down the tiled hallway, she managed a faint smile and exited without fanfare.

In magical fifteen-minute intervals for twenty-plus years, the drama has unfolded and replayed itself out on multiple stages in my practice and with a myriad of fascinating endings, both glorious and tragic. Every patient encounter has presented its own opportunities and challenges to heal and learn. When my soul becomes receptive, the spirits of past patients emerge and return to my collective consciousness to offer inspiration and much-needed guidance with difficult clinical situations.

In this arena young couples excitedly learned that they were pregnant with their first child, and vulnerable people received a tearful revelation that the candle of their lives was soon to be snuffed out. In foreboding medical territories such as cancer, dementia and chronic medical illness, it was tempting to feel helpless, with a bitter acknowledgement of defeat. Sometimes, all I could do was to offer emotional support and spiritual healing. When the doctor-patient process progressed smoothly, there was a mutual respect and shared appreciation: a prompt and correct diagnosis, a timely transfer of a critically ill patient to the ER, or a rapid necessary specialist consultation.

All too often things in the office didn't always go as planned. An angry patient and their family became confrontational about an actual or perceived misdiagnosis. Demanding people were steadfastly insistent on unnecessary antibiotic prescriptions, expensive medical tests, or unproven medical therapies. Dysfunctional families engaged in open conflict required my support and guidance in overwhelming situations with elusive solutions. Patients valiantly attempted to overcome significant economic and social barriers to access high-quality medical care. Sons and daughters, disconnected in a distant city, were harshly second-guessing how I was treating their elderly parent. Adverse situations such as these often led me to question my intelligence, competence, or worst of all, my humanity.

Family medicine encompasses everything about a patient. Like eager understudies, my fellow family physicians and I wait in the wings to assume an important dramatic medical role in the passion play of our patients' lives when most needed: obstetrician, psychiatrist, geriatrician, internist, pediatrician. We pride ourselves in being big-picture people and seeing our patients in their entirety, not a conglomeration of organ systems. As a family medicine doctor, I possess a unique opportunity to positively impact those around me in an incredibly gratifying manner on multiple levels. Equally humbling, I have had to acknowledge my human frailty and the sobering realization that I do not possess all of the answers desperately sought by my patients. I have grappled with the unpleasant reality of being equally capable of making mistakes and falling short of high expectations. All too often I have found myself wondering why I wanted to become a family physician in the first place, quickly dismissing it as a heresy.

After a busy morning I received a frantic phone call from the nursing home where I served as the medical director. One of my special patients, a kind eighty-two-year-old man from the independent living section named Bob Murphy, had an acute change in condition. He was lethargic, confused, and his blood pressure was frighteningly low at 80/50. My nurse practitioner in residence arranged an urgent ambulance transfer to our local hospital's emergency department. Mr. Murphy subsequently required admission into the intensive care unit, needing initial stabilization with appropriate medications and fluids. Bob was critically ill with sepsis, and I would need to revisit the hospital after office hours to assess his condition. Between the onrushing gauntlet of patients and rapid, sporadic bites of my lunch, I dutifully completed his orders and lined up the consultants to evaluate his multiple medical problems. I hoped that his blood pressure and medical status would improve as the afternoon progressed. It was shaping up to be a nutty day.

Office hours finally concluded, and I hunched over the counter at the nurses' station, reflectively looking down my hallway at the bank of now empty patient rooms. How did I get here? Being a family physician is an incredibly rewarding vocation, but often exhausting and challenging. My story didn't appear to be dramatic at first glance. I grew up in a small Iowa town, went to public schools, attended college and medical school at the nearby University of Iowa. My skill set with regard to scientific knowledge and training was solid, but in my mind seemed to pale in comparison to other students from elite prep schools and colleges around the country. Yet I had a Doctor of Medicine sheepskin hanging in my office and an M.D. monogrammed on to my white lab coat. My dedication to accumulating clinical expertise and perfecting my medical craft succeeded, and my career pathway took me to my dream job.

On the way to the hospital to see Mr. Murphy, I passed several budding corn and bean fields. Farmers on well-worn tractors were hard at work completing the spring planting process. I remembered my summer job during high school. My buddies and I spent June through August detasseling corn, the least favorite job I ever had in my entire life. To avoid undesired cross-pollination between corn plants, the yellow ornate tops of the corn stalks called tassels needed to be removed. It was hot and boring work. Early in the day, the corn plants were covered in dew and saturated our clothes as we walked through the fields to perform our menial labors. The leaves on the plants were rough, with a slight serration to them, which as they dried out over the day would scratch and irritate our forearms, especially if we forgot to wear a long-sleeve shirt. In the afternoon, the furnace-like heat and oppressive humidity of a July day would combine with heavy pollen-laden air to make breathing and moving miserable. Sometimes cars would pass us on the busy highway adjacent to the fields, tauntingly honk at us and make cruel remarks about our lot in life. I hated every minute of that job. Even though I was working with good friends, after my senior year of high school I vowed that I would never return to that godforsaken cornfield again.

With the passage of time, my negative recollection of that experience softened and evolved into a deeper understanding of growing from adversity. I thought about all of the high school kids across Iowa from my era who went through similar rites of passage, often with backbreaking, undesirable summer jobs, especially in agricultural communities. When we took the next educational steps into college, that previous unwelcome work ethic forcibly instilled in us served us well in our academic pursuits. In medical school, many of my native Iowan classmates and I shared these mutual life experiences, which propelled us through the difficulties of first-year bookwork and the onslaught of demanding third-year rotations. We emerged from our medical school training as accomplished graduate physicians, and through residency training programs nationwide we shared our Midwestern knowledge and values.

During growing season, most rural Iowans would obsess daily about the status of the agricultural situation. Was it too hot or too cold? Too much rain or not enough? Would there be a bumper crop or a drought? When I was eight years old, my great-grandmother always wanted to take a summertime drive out in the country after church services to check out how all the crops were doing. I slumped into the depths of the back seat, bored beyond comprehension. *These fields all look the same, Great-grandma! Just a bunch of corn, beans and alfalfa taking forever to grow!*

In the moment, it appeared to be a colossal waste of time, but its larger impact has now become apparent. My family recognized slight flaws in a field, where the corn or beans didn't look quite right, which could represent early disease and ultimately affect the harvest. Similarly, subtle patient clinical signs noted in the doctor's office can be a harbinger of more serious health issues. I reminisced and thought of all the hard work invested by the farmers in the spring planting season to ensure an annual successful yield. Under a nurturing sky, I cultivate my love and effort toward my seedling patients, hoping for a fruitful healthy harvest, knowing that there will always be variable times under every temperamental season—to be born and to die, to sow and to reap, to laugh and to weep. The undulating fields of joys and sorrows of life roll outward in all directions, *ad infinitum.*

Out of this fertile topsoil is where my journey begins.

CHAPTER 2

ROOTS

Midwestern roots, whether they are in a field or a family, tend to run deep and secure. My father was born on the Fourth of July, in 1938, always believing as a child that fireworks were a celebration of his birthday. He grew up happy and safe, unaware of the twin calamities of the Great Depression and the Second World War that enveloped the country. He was the youngest of four children, and after graduating from high school, enlisted in the United States Navy. Starting from Great Lakes Naval Base in suburban Chicago, his journeys took him to locations he only dreamt about or read in books: Rhode Island, the Mediterranean, Naples, Sicily, Athens, Istanbul. He returned home on leave stronger, more confident and, much to the consternation of his mother, adorned with multiple tattoos. He met and fell in love with my mother, and two years later they were married after his honorable discharge to his hometown of Oskaloosa, Iowa.

After working a few starter jobs at Gildner's Men's Store and a Kresge's Department Store, a hometown insurance agent named

Charles Brown took my dad under his wing and taught him to become an Independent Insurance Agent. Despite not having seized upon an opportunity to obtain a college education, my father grew and thrived in his new role. He immersed himself in the complexities of insurance underwriting, and mastered them with the level of proficiency of a college graduate. Subsequently, he twinned his newfound insurance expertise with an innate ability to relate to people from all walks of life. His clients appreciated his kind, ethical and honest approaches in their business dealings.

Like all parents, he was not free of the quirks that cause children to roll their eyes in exasperation. His tastes were simple and specific: Winston cigarettes, big Pontiac cars, and instant macaroni and cheese dinners. He was obscenely punctual in that being timely was actually ten minutes early, and arriving on time was considered tardy. He used the military term *pogey bait* to describe snacks between meals which could ruin my dinnertime appetite; he was always monitoring me to make sure I cleaned my plate. He detested big cities, crowds, and driving in congested levels of traffic, frequently avoiding grand events for his perception of personal comfort and security. We even disagreed about the correct way to mow our yard and perform repairs around the house.

When we weren't at odds with each other, my dad could be a powerful mentor to me while growing up in the bucolic serenity of a small Iowa town. At the beginning of my third summer in minor league baseball, I began to feel an increasing internal sense of frustration and inadequacy. While the other boys on my team improved their hitting, throwing and catching the ball compared to the last year, I seemed to be stuck in a rut. I dreaded the prospect of hanging out alone in right field during warm sun-drenched summer days, displaying my annual portrait of mediocrity. One mild late-April evening as I sat out on the back patio, despondently contemplating another long season on the diamond, my father came outside and joined me.

"Hey Bruce, what's goin' on? You seem quiet tonight."

"Yeah Dad, I'm just not looking forward to another baseball season, everyone on my team is getting better but me. I'm not going anywhere with baseball. Maybe I should try a different sport."

"Well, have you tried *practicing* at baseball on your own time at all?"

"Uh, no."

"How can you expect to grow and get better at something if you never put forth an effort to work on your skills? You know the league MVP from last year, Craig Lennox?"

Of course I remembered Craig. A legendary shortstop. Great fielding, a rocket arm and consistent hitting, an intelligent player. Literally, he was the complete package on the baseball field. Looked like he was born to play baseball from the minute he could hold a ball. "Sure, I remember him," I replied cautiously, uncertain of the direction of this conversation.

"Did you know that every spring he practices fielding with his dad, or playing pickup baseball with friends, or working on fundamentals nearly every night for about ninety minutes?"

"No, Dad, I didn't know that." It was hard for me to comprehend that such gifted athletes would invest a significant amount of personal capital perfecting their craft. In my myopic worldview, talented players received their abilities mysteriously without any impressive level of effort.

"Bruce, natural ability and talent only gets you so far in this world. What you lack in those areas you must make up for in hard work and determination. But you have to be committed to the process."

"Dad, can we work on these things so I can be ready for this baseball season?"

"Absolutely, I thought that you'd never ask."

"Why didn't you offer to help me out with this sooner?" I asked, somewhat exasperated that we should have worked on these things previously.

"You weren't mentally ready to practice and improve until now," Dad countered. "Once you displayed commitment to the work involved, then we could move forward."

Thus began a memorable summer season where I learned the importance of earnest engagement toward excellence. Natural abilities are helpful, yes, but I then realized an opportunity existed for cultivating previously unknown innate gifts. Throughout the remainder of the spring and early summer, every night after supper Dad and I would go out into the backyard and train in the fine arts of baseball skills. For well over an hour, with the fireflies joyously dancing all around us, we practiced catching, throwing and hitting. For the first time in my life, I genuinely enjoyed an athletic pursuit. I understood that I was going to get better, and I was receiving the gift of my father's guidance and attention through the precious interaction of a father-son catch game.

As the baseball season commenced, I became stronger and more athletic. In addition, I experienced a newfound sense of confidence in that my efforts were positively impacting myself and my teammates. My throwing arm was now quick and surprisingly accurate. I was hitting the ball with consistency and precision, and reaching base reliably and with regularity. Ultimately, my coaches noticed my work ethic and vastly improved skill set. Seemingly overnight, I was moved from right field obscurity to the bustling shortstop position, my first time ever playing in the infield. The magical season climaxed with my game-winning hit to advance to the championship game and being selected to the All-Star Team. Many summers later, I have never forgotten the significance of that special baseball season, with its treasured father-son time resulting in a brief athletic renaissance.

My father-in-law Jim is an incredibly talented handyman. He has never had any formal training or apprenticeship in the trades, but his depth of knowledge is on a par with many skilled craftsmen. His organized and orderly approach to solving problems is admirable, and results in an ideal, functional solution: a repaired light socket, a well-painted wall, or a properly aligned cabinet door. I attempt to absorb every insightful handy tidbit he graciously shares. These concepts have been useful, not only for home improvement issues, but also refining my style for diagnosing and treating my patients so that they feel rejuvenated and happy.

Several years ago, Jim took on a self-starting home improvement project that was quite ambitious, even for him: constructing a deck off of the back of his house. This was not to be an ordinary deck; rather, it was planned to be a two-level affair, built into a sloping hill that fell away from the house in every direction imaginable. The design called for ornate handrails and a protective synthetic veneer-surfaced superstructure. Warily and with healthy skepticism, I watched as he deliberately outlined the concept for the project, with self-drawn and carefully crafted plans. I was uncertain if he realized the true demands of such an audacious undertaking.

With the proposed design completed, materials ordered and delivered, and concrete support piers poured into the ground, it was time to get to the heart of the work. Jim, his son Jim Jr. and I walked out to the backyard on a warm spring morning and surveyed the monumental task that lay ahead of us. With a simple "OK, let's go" from Papa Jim, we determinedly embarked on our hard day's work project. For hours the three of us labored under the warm, glorious sunshine and gentle swirling breezes. With deliberate precision we erected the base supports, followed by the heavy, massive joists that took all of our collective strength to maneuver and secure into place. More than once, I found myself questioning my fitness and endurance, as well as the feasibility of this project. My upper-body muscles and legs ached with ever-increasing soreness. Jim made eye contact with me in the heat of the moment and innately sensed my pessimism and concern.

"Hey Bruce, keep up the good work, we're making great progress, thanks to you. I know it's hard to believe, but this project will look amazing once it's finished."

"OK Jim, I trust you. Let me know what you need me to do."

Once the supplemental joists and supports were interlocked with a steadily coalescing superstructure, Jim's confident prophecy was proven correct. The graceful deck frame hugged the rear of the house and extended over the backyard hill, exactly how Jim visualized it. Throughout the afternoon, like focused busy worker bees, the three of us screwed sections of floorboard onto the underlying joists and frame areas. I banished all negative thoughts about the project to the deep recesses of my collective consciousness. By 5:30 p.m., the wooden portion of the project was completed. It was time for a couple of beers and a celebration of a job well done. For several summers thereafter we enjoyed the fruits of our labor on that deck with delicious libations and lively conversation.

As I drove back to Milwaukee happily exhausted and with an exuberant sense of accomplishment, my thoughts went back to Jim and his amazing achievement. How did he possess the intelligence to complete such a complicated undertaking? Where did his methodical approach to problem-solving germinate and bloom? When I pointedly asked him this question, his response was simple: "My father and father-in-law taught me all that I needed to know for home improvement projects." Thus his knowledge was acquired simply and not mystically, in the recurrent oral and demonstrative tradition of his ancestors. He eloquently summarized the pedagogical approach to development in any vocation, especially medicine: *Watch, listen and learn, perfect your skills, then teach your insight and experiences to the younger generation.* Whether educating a budding young physician assistant student or trying to stay current with journal articles and medical conferences, I think about how Jim served as my role model for being both a good student and an inspiring mentor.

In medicine, just as often mentoring can unexpectedly emanate from someone who demonstrates what *not* to do in patient care approaches. As a third-year medical student, I was busy on a surgical subspecialty service. We spent long hours every day operating, checking in on hospital patients, and completing bustling sessions in the outpatient clinic. One particularly hectic office day, I was excited to hear that Dr. Monroe, the chairman of the department, was supervising the clinic. His intellect, surgical skills and reputation were the source of international renown. I looked forward to him sharing some of his cutting-edge medical knowledge with me, and hopefully establish a professional connection in case I needed a reference for a residency position some day.

Finally, in the middle of a chaotic clinic morning, the time arrived to present a case to Dr. Monroe. We moved the patient to a special exam room which directly adjoined Dr. Monroe's office and was for his use only. The first-year resident, well aware of my enthusiasm and inquisitive spirit on this rotation, took me aside and preemptively gave me a stern admonishment:

"Bruce—follow my lead when we go in to present the case to Dr. Monroe. No eye contact with the chief, no small talk, no medical questions, *no nothing* . . . got it?"

"Yes, Dr. Jacobs, I understand and I promise to be on my best behavior," I replied courteously, now curious as to what all the hubbub was about for this particular program chair.

My resident crisply knocked on the chief's door exactly three times, and upon hearing a deadpan "come in," methodically walked into the immense office and toward Dr. Monroe's desk. I tried my best to emulate my senior resident's mannerisms in the most uniform manner possible so as to not draw attention to myself.

Dr. Jacobs exchanged no greetings with the chief. There were no smiles, shared pleasantries or small talk between the two. I might as well not even existed—third-year medical students should not be seen *nor* heard. *Wow, I can't believe he's completely ignoring me . . . so much for the residency reference.* My first-year resident placed the patient's chart precisely on the right front corner of the massive ornate mahogany desk and with eyes focused straight forward, began his mechanical presentation. "Mrs. Humphrey is a forty-seven-year-old white female with a history of progressive abdominal pain over the last several weeks . . ."

While the first-year outlined in methodical detail the medical soliloquy, I struggled mightily to keep my eyes straight ahead, attempting to ignore the innumerable diplomas and awards that covered every available inch of the walls. Out of the corner of my peripheral vision I cheated a few glances at Dr. Monroe. The gray-haired famous chief sat emotionless, looked downward on to the highly polished desk, nodding his head and grunting after every few spoken sentences. I had envisioned a much different first encounter with the world-renowned doctor who had guided the department to become one of the top-ranked programs in the nation. After a few minutes of presenting, he abruptly raised his right hand to indicate that he had heard enough.

"OK—let's go see this lady," he answered blandly.

We followed him into his personalized exam room where he could assess Mrs. Humphrey. The coldness of emotions and minimalist social interaction extended to the patient visit. "Hi, I'm Dr. Monroe," he simply said. There was no smile, handshake, sharing of a laugh or emotion, or establishing rapport like we were taught in our Introduction to Clinical Medicine class. The frigidity and lack of empathy seemed to envelop the surroundings. Mrs. Humphrey was polite and serious, doing her part not to disrupt the great doctor. Dr. Monroe completed a brief examination, and turning to the resident, issued a few sparse instructions for the patient's treatment. Unexpectedly, the chief departed the room without so much as a goodbye. Our patient was not asked whether she had any questions, understood her diagnosis, or agreed with her care plan. My resident finished with Mrs. Humphrey, trying to fill in the gaping holes of information and emotional void left by our illustrious leader. A few minutes later, she left and the bizarre visit concluded.

What the hell was that? I thought quizzically. This guy is one of the best doctors in his field—in the nation, maybe even the world. He had taught countless practicing physicians, conducted groundbreaking research, and was highly respected by every program chair at the University Hospital and far beyond its beige walls. Almost every department in the country would have loved to have him serve as their program chairman. But all I felt was disappointment in one of my perceived role models, and maybe even some level of pity for him. He was missing out on an entirely spectacular aspect of medicine. Yes, it was a tremendous blessing and rewarding to be intelligent, technically gifted and respected by peers. It is *also* hugely important to possess the emotional intelligence to read a patient's nonverbal cues and enter into meaningful therapeutic relationships.

I promised myself from that moment forward that I would socially interact with a patient differently from the Dr. Monroe style. I always start patient visits with a handshake and a smile, small talk and set an empathetic stage for each encounter.

It was early summer, and my family was enjoying a lovely week in Wisconsin on the Door County Peninsula. We escaped the unusual June heat wave with an excursion to Lake Michigan and the Cana Island Lighthouse. The inland coast was windswept and moderately cooler, with a steady lake breeze emanating from the perennially chilled depths of the Great Lakes waters. The stony beach was bathed in sunlight, intermittently obscured by puffy cumulus clouds lazily strolling above us.

Carefully we traversed an irregular, rocky causeway out to the lighthouse and the keeper's quarters. As I stood under the towering and tapering whitish metallic structure, I marveled at its endurance to withstand the myriad of storms and changing conditions through the years, as well as guiding the generations of mariners who have sailed along its hazardous shores. My thoughts turned to my father, my father-in-law Jim and the countless teachers who have guided me, with both positive and negative life lessons. Like the solitary, resilient lighthouse, I hoped that my life would serve as a guiding light to others, providing safe passage from the hazards of insecurity and ignorance.

CHAPTER 3

IMPRESSIONS

In the business world, social circles and even medicine, first impressions have powerful impacts upon relationships, success and formulating diagnoses. On many occasions, this insight is helpful: It allows me to see through a patient unintentionally presenting confusing historical information, or a physical exam finding that doesn't fit with the rest of the clinical picture. Due to the experience and confidence developed over many years of clinical practice, I can arrive at a provisional diagnosis quickly. When I am able to "figure it out" during a clinic visit, it has the added bonus of bolstering some patient confidence in me: *He made the right diagnosis, rapidly treated me and I got better. I am lucky to have him as my doctor.* Similarly, the outward intangible picture that I present to others is important as well—an earnest smile, confident handshake, colorful bow tie and thoughtful eye contact have served me well in thousands of clinical interactions.

This tryout was going to be huge. Our high school was scheduled to put on the musical *You're a Good Man, Charlie Brown*, and given the small nature of the cast, only a few parts were available. Even in a small-town Iowa high school, the annual musical is quite the dramatic extravaganza. However, this year the director was taking a calculated risk in that even with our relatively solid school talent pool, we would be best served by a smaller, high-talented cast as opposed to the typical "cast of thousands" which are frequent hallmarks of many musical ensembles.

It was a venture that caused me some discomforting feelings. By this juncture, I was a sophomore in high school, and a veteran of many local theater productions. However, I had never previously auditioned for a high school theatrical show, and based on seniority I was one of the lower life-forms in the high school hallway habitat. I became determined not to allow my social self-consciousness discourage me from trying out for one of the nine leading parts in the show.

On first glance, the talent pool appeared to be daunting: multiple juniors and seniors, boys and girls alike, with strong voices and commanding stage presence; and to my surprise, aspiring sophomores and even a few enthusiastic freshmen eager to add their artistic skills to the ensemble. I had about two weeks to prepare material, practice and refine my singing numbers, expressively read a few lines of choice dialogue, and figure out how to interact with my fellow actors with appropriate chemistry and energy. When taken as a whole, the project workload seemed to be overwhelming, a task that could ultimately prove to be impossible to master. As the tryouts drew near, however, I began to develop a growing sense of confidence that my natural artistic talents and hard work would hold my own with my older and perhaps more-gifted counterparts.

Auditions for theatrical productions were always a fascinating experience. Often the window of opportunity in a tryout is brief. For this session, I read a few passages for Linus, Snoopy and Charlie Brown. Then I practiced dialogue with someone playing a complementary character. The director remained stonefaced, but my optimism steadily increased and blossomed as I began to be called back up on multiple occasions to read more lines with various configurations of characters, most of them juniors and seniors. *Could it be that I actually have an inside track on this thing? Are they that interested in me right now? I have a pretty loud and projecting voice, so they are probably just using me so that the others may practice their lines and get their inflections and volumes set up properly.* Still, I continued to carry myself with youthful enthusiasm and self-assurance in the hopes of securing a role in this competitive production.

It was time for us to sing a number from the musical, so that the choir director could get a sense of our vocalization quality. Normally this was always one of my strong suits, but a funny thing began to happen to me last summer, a common childhood phenomenon known as puberty. As a result, my typically pristine high tenor-low alto voice had morphed into a warbling mid-tenor sound, with occasional breaks in continuity and a squeaky vocal inconsistency to which I was not accustomed. Fortunately, I had used the last couple of weeks practicing techniques with my choir director to help smooth over the rough edges and jumpy contours to my vocal pattern.

At last, the time had arrived for me to complete my tryout by singing a short selection, a thirty- to sixty-second single shot at secondary school theatrical greatness. As I stood solitarily on the stage, and heard the choral director bang out the introductory chords to my piece, I felt the wobbly sensation in my legs lessen, the tightness in my chest and throat steadily diminish, then relinquish itself completely. *I worked hard to get here. I deserve this opportunity for a part in this great show. My abilities and gifts can stand up among the best people here in this room.* After completing my last thought, my cue arrived and I began to sing confidently, without any awkward pubescent breaks in my vocal register. I was doing it, and maximizing this chance afforded to me in a tight one-minute performance slot. The selection concluded, and I felt a great sense of pride regarding my singing display while relieved that the stressful tryout ordeal was over. I smiled as I heard a formal and curt "Thank you" from the two directors and, cliche-like, I exited stage right.

My two-block walk home from the high school was filled with serenity, as I jauntily sang many of the songs I had practiced from the show. I quietly dreamed that I would perform them again as a part of a quality high school production. Two days later, I was overjoyed and honored as my efforts were rewarded with the part of Linus. I recognized the power of twinning first impressions and self-confidence in order to positively present myself to the outside world and achieve a goal which I desperately wanted.

Veronica was a delightful, forty-five-year-old married mother of two who had been a patient in my medical practice for many years. A few years ago, we needed to hospitalize her for an attack of acute diverticulitis, an infection of the lining of her colon. The diagnosis was easily made, and she responded to a short hospital stay with IV antibiotics. Several months later, she returned to my office with a complaint of recurrent abdominal pain. This reflected a dilemma that often confronts clinicians: Patient has a problem for many years with recurrent symptoms and presentation, and is explained by a traditional, specific diagnosis, let's call it Diagnosis A. Every time that this person sees us in the office with these same collection of symptoms, will it always be Diagnosis A, or this time will it be a different diagnosis? It is critically important for doctors to avoid rushing to conclusions, assuming the same repetitive problem is always taking place.

"Hi Veronica, what's goin' on with your belly pain?"

"Well, Dr. Rowe, it started about three days ago, and it's all over my stomach. Maybe it was something we ate, but no one else got sick."

"How bad is it—can you give it a number on a scale from 1 to 10? What's it feel like?"

"It feels like a dull ache, about a 7 out of 10, not in one specific place."

"Is it worse down on the lower left side, like it was last time?" Left lower quadrant abdominal pain is the classic presenting region in the setting of diverticulitis.

"I'm not sure, it kinda hurts all over today."

"Any nausea or vomiting, blood in the stool, or vomiting up blood?"

"No, except maybe just a little nausea."

Then I asked a seemingly routine, but revealing question: "Does the pain move anywhere?"

A moment of clarity and a crucial comment from the patient: "Why yes, I get a pain around my belly button that shoots straight through to my back. That's happened a few times recently."

That type of pain and presentation is often diagnostic of a specific medical problem: pancreatitis, usually due to alcohol or gallstones. Veronica had never had any previous abdominal surgeries and was an occasional drinker, so this potential diagnosis was a very viable one. On physical examination her pain seemed to be localized over the belly button area, where she described the worst of her affliction. After only a few minutes of history taking and questions, a realistic cause and targeted solution appeared to be crystallizing into place.

"Veronica, I think you may have gallstone pancreatitis, a problem where gallstones get stuck in the bile duct and inflame the pancreas. It sometimes can be a serious issue. I don't know for sure, but we should get some blood work and an ultrasound of your gallbladder and pancreas."

"Really? You can figure all of that out just by talking to me for a few minutes and feeling around on my belly?"

"I know it seems weird, but we see these things a lot in practice, and based on your description, the pattern fits with other patients that have had this problem."

I paused for a moment to contemplate in my head what I was saying out loud. *Patterns? Am I drawing from experience, or am I risking erroneously pigeonholing my patient and her diagnosis?* Medical pattern recognition based on solid, complete first impressions can be a great asset if used carefully at the patient's bedside.

"OK Dr. Rowe, I trust you, you've never steered me wrong before. Let's get the testing done today."

Veronica's lab work showed significantly elevated levels of amylase and lipase, around 1000 for each lab—normal level is less than 50. This was diagnostic of acute pancreatitis. The elevated liver function tests, coupled with the ultrasound which showed rocky shadows and a dilated common bile duct, confirmed that the pancreatitis was gallstone in origin and not related to alcohol or medications. A few days later the stones were removed from the duct and her gallbladder extracted. She made a great recovery and is doing well today. I felt a deep sense of satisfaction that within a framework of clinical experience and initial impressions I was able to synthesize medical history, examination and lab tests to effectively diagnose and treat my patient.

However, for every gut-instinct victory, with healing and happy patients, there are the curveballs, ones that humble me and potentially place my patients in jeopardy. With alarming frequency in medicine, first impressions can be misleading and may result in a delayed diagnosis, treatment deviations and, unfortunately, serious and perhaps even fatal outcomes. Overconfidence and and false clarity can result in inappropriate assumptions, a rush down an incorrect clinical pathway toward inaccurate conclusions, threatening the patient's well-being, and casting the physician in quite an unflattering light. Too often I get down on myself when the patient visit goes wrong—frequently I have questioned my knowledge, wondered whether I pressed the visit, was too busy or distracted to hear that all-important piece of clinical information. There is a significant amount of stress and soul-searching that these cases can engender in a young doctor. Case situations where false preconceptions placed me on the wrong diagnostic track were some of the most effective learning experiences that I have encountered.

For my first week as a resident, I found myself on an inpatient internal medicine service in Waukesha, Wisconsin. My fellow resident had an interesting patient that she lovingly nicknamed Crazy Eleanor. She had too many possessions and cats in her home, and always seemed to be on the verge of not being able to live independently because of various physical and mental issues. She frequented our office with many medical complaints which seemed difficult to sort out and bordered on hypochondriasis. However, she also displayed cases of true medical illness and required stays in the hospital for a variety of ailments: a bout of pneumonia, a right hip fracture, or an acute episode of dehydration. My partner pleasantly talked of her idiosyncrasies and the adventures of figuring out her latest medical malady and helping her to work through her adversity. So I wasn't terribly surprised to receive a phone call from the ED on a warm summer Sunday evening notifying me of the need to admit Eleanor to the hospital. She arrived with a fever, elevated white blood cell count, and a urinalysis full of bacteria.

I examined Eleanor and placed some orders for her hospitalization for an acute urinary tract infection. However, early on it appeared that something didn't seem quite right. I had never met Crazy Eleanor before, but she didn't seem like she was the person that my colleague Kathy had positively talked about in conversation. First of all, she was not pleasant nor quirky—in fact, she seemed agitated and didn't want to answer any questions. In addition, she was increasingly confused and unaware of her surroundings. Our conversation was circuitous and did very little to accomplish clarification of her medical issues.

"Now Eleanor, if you can tell me when you started feeling like—"

"Where's my kitty? Where's Ollie? He must be hiding! He needs to be fed. Be a dear and fetch his food out of the fridge, will you?"

"Eleanor, you're not at home, you're in the hospital. Have you noticed any foul odor or pain with your urin—"

"Don't lie to me about my kitty! We need to find him, stop asking me all these silly questions . . ."

I became convinced during our interaction that she was developing some degree of progressive dementia, and she would require some long-term care arrangement. I abandoned any hope of obtaining any semblance of a patient history. The physical examination was normal with the exception of some mild lower abdominal tenderness over her urinary bladder. Finally, I completed her admissions paperwork, began her on some IV antibiotics and IV fluids, ordered labs for the morning and went to bed.

The following morning, I presented Crazy Eleanor's case to my inpatient service team. Rounding in teaching hospitals occurs as a group so that we can get to know about all of the patients on the service together. During my succinct case presentation I indicated my significant worries about Eleanor's decline in mentation and my belief that we should consult discharge planning for a possible nursing home placement. Wrapping up the discussion of treatment plans and the day's goals outside of Eleanor's room, I prepared to be vindicated.

At this point things began to get interesting. As I led my attending doctor and fellow residents into Eleanor's room, I immediately realized that everything with her health situation had completely turned upside down compared to last evening, and nothing was what it had seemed to be yesterday. Eleanor wasn't angry or agitated or confused anymore. In fact, she was smiling and conversant.

"Oh good morning, Doctors!" she chirped happily. "I'm just finishing up my breakfast, and I feel so much better today. In fact, I don't even remember what happened last night."

Now I felt embarrassed and foolish. I had presented a case and a situation in which I was confident of her diagnosis and her outcome: urinary tract infection (UTI) and progressive dementia. We had treated her UTI; did we "cure" her dementia in the process? The entire scenario was not making sense, and I felt like I was attempting to solve a jigsaw puzzle with an incomplete set of component pieces. I struggled to maintain my composure and salvage the remainder of my insight and plan.

"She wasn't looking this good last night . . . I mean she was sick and confused when I admitted her, and I seriously thought she wasn't going to be able to return back home."

Dr. Jay Friedman, my attending physician, looked at me with a pleasant smile. "Bruce, you fixed her. She had a case of delirium—acute mental confusion most likely brought on by her urinary tract infection. It should resolve completely without any long-term effects. Now that the antibiotics and the fluids have kicked in, she should make a full recovery and be able to go home in a few days. You'll see this problem countless times in medical practice, especially in the elderly; this was just the first time that you encountered it. Got that, everybody?" I could tell by the looks on my empathetic fellow residents' faces that they had either previously been through this experience or were learning from my example.

As I walked out to my car that night, I felt humbled and chastened, but also encouraged. I learned that first impressions can be important, but so is thoughtful, deliberate thinking to arrive at the correct diagnosis. I promised myself that I would be careful to balance these two competing approaches as a practicing physician.

It was freshman year at the University of Iowa, and a common rite of passage for the engineers and premeds was the *Introduction to Calculus* class. Our teacher my first fall was Dr. Ben Goodman, a gregarious, white-bearded sixty-something-year-old gentleman, always adorned with his favorite Detroit Tigers baseball cap. The course was interesting, informative and even entertaining. While I did very well in this competitive class, I could not help but be pleasantly distracted by one of my lovely classmates. I saw her walk in to class the first week, her mid-length wavy chestnut hair gently gracing her shoulders. She radiated happiness and confidence, and attracted friendly interactions everywhere that she went. Through my friends, I found out that her name was Laura.

We finally met in class and had a pleasant interaction, but it was purely of a platonic nature. While contemplating my next move, I learned that she was originally from the affluent Chicago suburbs, and was active in the leadership of her sorority chapter. As a small-town Iowa boy, a dorm geek not involved with Greek life, I felt my opportunity to expand my relationship with Laura diminish. *I mean, how could this ever work? Look at her life compared to mine . . . she is so smart, attractive, successful and supremely confident. I could never compete with that. What could I possibly have to offer her?*

With that grim premature first impression, I resigned myself to a friendly, distant relationship with Laura, but as the college years progressed I would see her occasionally. I continued to admire her from afar and never gave up hope that someday I would be able to overcome my lack of confidence and perceived differences to ultimately become more than just a friend to her. Only time and my personal efforts to shape myself into the type of person that I would want to be would complete the final chapters in the hopeful, ideal love story. I had no idea what the future held for me in terms of love; but I knew that if I was ever to win over Laura, it would take a series of positive impacts, carefully crafted to define myself as a person of talent, excellence and moral kindness. It appeared daunting and futile on the surface, but for this rural Iowa boy the effort to achieve true love was worth the reward. With that inspirational thought, I threw myself in to my schoolwork, increased my efforts in to self-improvement on all levels . . . and tried to put Laura out of my mind for the foreseeable future.

CHAPTER 4

VALLEY

My dad died very early in the chilled, desolate hours of a December Saturday morning. He was only fifty-one years old. Looking back, I should have seen it coming. He had sneakily resumed his smoking habit, not a well-kept secret given the obvious malodorous tobacco scent present on his clothes and in his car. In addition, his weight had ballooned by thirty pounds in two years, and after dinner every night he lazily relegated himself to his recliner to watch his favorite police detective shows. It was not a merciful passing or a valedictory heartfelt adieu to a long, beautiful life well lived. Rather, the events of that night were sudden, violent and heart wrenching, and left deep horrifying scars inscribed on the souls of everyone who was unfortunate enough to experience it.

On the Friday evening before the fateful day, I was in my dorm room in Iowa City, doing laundry and preparing for the looming finals week, then returning home for Winter Break. As a senior in the engineering school, it would be another challenging five days of testing. I took comfort in that I had only one more finals week as an undergraduate, and I had already been accepted early decision to medical school. It was glorious news, and my parents were so proud of me, a true high point in my life. On the car ride home with my father for what later proved to be our last Thanksgiving together, he said something heartfelt:

"Bruce, when I was a medic in the Navy, I loved medicine, but because I never worked hard I couldn't become a doctor. I'm so proud of this opportunity because of your hard work, but most importantly, I'm honored to call you my son." For my dad, this was a rare openness of emotions and baring of his soul.

"Thanks Dad—I promise I'll do my best in medical school, make you and Mom proud of me, and I won't let you down." My sacrifices had paid off, and a major career goal had been achieved.

Now just two weeks later, that fragile contentment was in the process of being shattered on this cold, eerily calm December evening. As I was getting my books and laundry detergent organized, the wall phone jangled loudly with a surreal sound of urgency. My roommate Jason picked up the phone, looked perplexed and then gently handed me the phone and said, "Here, it's for you . . . it's your mom . . . seems weird to be calling this late on a Friday night."

I nervously took the receiver, and after a greeting, listened as my upset, nearly hysterical mother summarized the events of the evening. "Your father got chest pains putting up the Christmas tree . . . drove him to the emergency room . . . is having a severe heart attack . . . shocked him back from the dead twice . . . Life-Flighted to Des Moines . . . has about a fifty-fifty chance of survival." Any single one of those phrases in that group of information would have been horrible by itself. Strung together in sequence like grim pearls, they formed a tragic chain of despair.

"OK Mom, I'm coming to Des Moines now, Jason said he'll drive me."

"Thanks Bruce. Monica is staying with Grandma. I'll meet you there at Mercy Hospital, please hurry, I don't know what is going to happen next." She lost her composure and began to cry as she hung up the phone.

It was now 11:00 p.m., and Jason, my friend Mike and I set off on a dark, bitterly cold evening on the due-westerly two-hour trek to Des Moines. It was an eerily quiet journey, and I feared the worst. As I slumped down in the front passenger seat, I fervently prayed to God to have mercy and save my father to live through this night. Nearing the eastern suburbs of the capital city, I felt the chilling sensation that my father had already left me for good. Around 1:00 a.m. we pulled into the hospital parking lot and took the elevator up to the fifth floor, the Cardiovascular ICU. The doors briskly opened, and I did not see my mom, but my dad's dear friend Bill approached me reluctantly. He looked shell-shocked and wore the saddest expression that I had ever witnessed. My emotional intelligence told me that something terrible had happened; to what severity I was about to find out.

"I'm so sorry, Bruce, but your dad passed away about forty-five minutes ago."

I felt my emotional floor give way as I saw myself hurtling uncontrollably into the darkest void. Time seemed to stand still as I felt a black hole of tragedy contracting at the speed of light upon my soul until compressed into a terrifying, awful singularity.

While I struggled to process this horrific piece of information, my mom suddenly appeared from around the corner. She looked blindsided and shattered, and seemed to have aged ten years overnight. I ran to her, filled with fear and vulnerability, the two of us horribly exposed to the harsh elements of a cruel world. After a protracted and heartbreaking embrace, through the tears I attempted the awkward balancing act of projecting strength to my mom, but needing comfort and support from her in return. *How could this have happened to us? What are we going to do?*

Dr. McGuiness, a pleasant middle-aged man, was the cardiologist on call that evening for Mercy Hospital. He took my mom and me to a quiet conference room and explained how the horror story unfolded.

"Well, first of all, I want to say how sorry I am for your loss. I cannot even comprehend what it must be like to lose your husband and father so tragically, and at such a young age. When Larry arrived here, he was in cardiogenic shock, and was incredibly unstable. At the local hospital, he had received streptokinase, a medication designed to break up blood clots in the coronary artery. Clearly, he was not responding to this intervention. We emergently took him back to the cardiac catheterization lab, where we found that all three of his major coronary arteries were severely diseased and almost completely blocked. He was bleeding internally from the streptokinase and was too deep in shock with low blood pressures to undergo emergency cardiac bypass surgery. As we were preparing to place a pump in the aorta to assist the heart, stabilize him and the blood pressure situation, he vomited large amounts of blood and went into cardiac arrest for a third time. Unfortunately, this time we were unable to save him. Again, I am so sorry for what happened, we really did all that we possibly could."

As my head was spinning, all I could ask was, "Were there any collateral branches between the coronaries that could have bought him some time?" Collateral blood vessels are generated by the body to create alternate routes to naturally bypass blocked areas.

"Sorry to say, Bruce, but very little of that was present, and then when the blockages reached a critical level, we quickly found out that he was in real trouble."

"OK, thanks, Doctor," I replied meekly.

"Did you guys have any other questions that I could answer for you this morning?" Dr. McGuiness kindly inquired. *Morning? Holy shit, that's right, it's like 2:00 a.m. now.*

"No, not right now, I'm just having a real hard time trying to process it all," Mom replied with unsettling resignation.

"I can't even comprehend what you guys are going through. Here is my card, if you have any further concerns over the coming weeks and months, please don't hesitate to give me a call. Again, I am so sorry about what happened . . ."

With the utmost of superhuman effort I attempted to show a brave face, and project some measure of strength as I shook the doctor's hand. "Thanks for all of your efforts and dedication here tonight," I replied, now with a more confident voice. "I know that you and your team gave it your best shot."

"You're welcome, Bruce . . . would you like to spend some time alone with your father for a few minutes?"

"Yes—I would like that very much."

The medical team respectfully brought me into the ICU room where my father lay in a tragic, quiet repose. Although things had been tidied up a bit, clear residual evidence of an epic futile battle to save a life remained. Around the room the agonizing chill of death was everywhere. A pall of doom tangibly exuded from the ordinary beige-colored walls and permeated my soul. Dad looked completely lifeless, his facial expression permanently etched in an unspeakable anguish depicting his last moments of life. I touched his body gently at first, then I gave him a heartfelt hug. The progressive total body stiffness of rigor mortis was already making its presence felt. *I never even got to say goodbye to him.* For twenty minutes I kept a lonely vigil, relating a hapless soliloquy, hoping that his spirit still remained in the vicinity. Through a veil of tears and occasional prism of anger I highlighted our short, pleasant life together.

"Dad, I know you can hear me. I can't believe that you're gone. I feel so lost, and I'm scared about what's going to become of our family. Thanks for being a great father. Please watch over us. I promise to take good care of Mom and Monica, and I'll make you proud. I will forever miss you, always love you, and never forget you."

Almost on cue, there was a gentle knock at the door, followed by the entrance of my mom and a sweet, sympathetic middle-aged Catholic nun.

"Hi Bruce, I am Sister Mary Margaret," she introduced herself with warmth and kindness. "Would it help your family feel a little measure of comfort to pray together?"

"Yes, please," I replied humbly, feeling insignificant in comparison to the uncontrolled cruel machinations of my surrounding universe.

The three of us joined hands in an intimate triangulated circle of support. "Dear Lord Jesus," she began solemnly, "please accept the soul of Larry into your blessed kingdom, and bless his widow Sandy, his son Bruce and his daughter Monica. We ask that you provide comfort and hope to his family in the days, weeks and months ahead. All of this we pray in the name of the Father, Son and Holy Spirit, Amen."

With that final amen, my mom and I departed Mercy Hospital, went out into the cold, snowy dark early-morning hours, started our painful exodus toward home, and began an excruciating venture toward an uncertain future.

The subsequent days leading up to the funeral seemed to pass by in an incomprehensible blur. I felt as if I was outside of my body, serving as a passive spectator to the unpleasant series of events. There was a continuous chain of well-wishers arriving at our modest house for days, a refrigerator filled to the point of bursting with home-cooked meals, mountains of cards and endless flowers, Mom's friends performing nonstop laundry, housework and greeting guests. Seeing all of my dad's friends, relatives and work associates as upset as me did provide a bizarre camaraderie of mutual suffering.

Wednesday, the day of the funeral, was sunny and clear, but fittingly ended up being the coldest day in December that year. At the graveside ceremony, in a hopeful yet futile attempt at a final terrestrial connection, I placed my hand on the top of the dark-brown walnut casket, leaving a moist handprint of condensation interlaced with the scarlet holly berries and dark-green thorny leaves of the holiday-themed holly casket spray. Within a few moments of removing my hand, the fragile moist imprint faded away, ephemeral, just like all human life.

As we laid my dad to rest in the beautiful quiet of Evergreen Cemetery west of town, and the residual cortege made its way back to the church for a late luncheon, some concerning realities were becoming apparent. I realized that finals week at my university was going on right now, and I was going to need to make up my exams. Already I could sense that the remainder of the world would not stop for long to mourn my father; soon life would resume its metronomic procession, regardless of my level of engagement in the process.

Ruthlessly, over the coming weeks, beyond Christmas into the new year, my depressing prophecy that I had made about human nature began to be fulfilled. Our friends, neighbors and relatives began to inevitably return to their own lives and existences. The phone calls, cards and spontaneous invitations to various activities began to dry up. It wasn't that our fellow townspeople didn't care about us; we knew that they continued to love and pray for our family. The simple truth is that life is for the living, and ultimate human behavior is to enjoy life to the fullest. It takes a tremendous amount of time and energy to maintain an anxious, fear-ridden grieving process. The world had paid its tribute to my father, but like every other tragic loss throughout the millennia, humanity had recorded his beautiful but brief eulogistic history and turned the page. The challenge presented to me was to balance a culture of honoring the memory of my father while positively moving forward.

Over the succeeding months, with a nagging spiritual void I completed my undergraduate degree, but graduation day felt hollow without my father in attendance. After an all-too-quick summer break, it was time to return to Iowa City for the quadrennial exercise in educational and emotional endurance called medical school. Suddenly I found myself in a large auditorium with 174 of my fellow classmates from all around the state of Iowa, throughout the country, and from all conceivable walks of life. Everyone was excited, nervous and filled with uncertainty and anticipation about what the next four years would hold.

Almost immediately I felt the pressure and struggle to keep up with an ever-oncoming avalanche of facts and concepts to master and memorize, all in an intensive incubator of academic development where everyone in the class was as intelligent and dedicated as me. The glaring exception was that compared to my energized and focused classmates, I felt at a bit of a disadvantage. While studying late into the evening, I thought of my dad and in my grief would contemplate, *What's the point of this? All I know is that my dad is no longer around, and I feel incomplete and broken.* My classmates' parents, typically a happy and intact mother and father unit, would frequently come and visit them on the weekends. I found myself jealous and bitterly resenting their cohesive, loving family structures, happiness and upper-middle-class standard of living. I am amazed that I got through the journey at all. A lot of people helped me cross over that foreboding collegiate mountain pass to graduation. My mom wrote me inspiring letters, my roommate Jason kept my spirits up with jokes and encouragement, and internally I willed myself to succeed because my father and I dreamed about my ultimate career in medicine.

Divine inspiration and salvation arrived during a special and momentous fall of my second year of medical school through unlikely venues. All second-years were required to take a class called

Systemic Pathology, a comprehensive, demanding class that took us through every organ system of the body, meticulously identifying normal function and disease states. It was hard, with challenging amounts of detailed clinical information, and I loved every minute of it. For the first time in well over a year, I felt an intellectual fire burning inside the core of my being. Disease processes were complicated, infinite in presentation and scope, and above all else . . . interesting. I experienced a sensation of stepping over a threshold, from a dark past into a bright future. *I can do this! I have what it takes! It's not just all about rote memorization of a huge cadre of facts and figures! Now we get to diagnose and heal patients! Yes!* From that class onward, I once again believed that I belonged in medical school with my classmates, that all along I had all the skills that I needed to succeed in my medical training process.

On an October Friday night, my buddies and I were at a medical fraternity party. As we procured our bathtub gin drinks I turned and saw her—she was radiant, smiling, with a shorter, light-brown haircut. I knew who she was all along, and the pleasant memories rapidly returned. As an undergrad, while I hung out with my dorm buddies, she was a sorority/Greek-life-based leader, well-liked by everyone on campus. Back then, I was too shy to pursue a relationship, and had resigned myself to admiration from a distance. At this juncture, however, the circumstances had changed: She was a grad student in speech pathology, while I had obtained my engineering degree and was now well into my medical school training. My confidence and sense of purpose over the intervening years had grown and been rejuvenated. It was my first college crush, and seeing her again was a delightful surprise. I saw her smiling at me and moving in my direction. *Holy crap! What do I do now?*

"Hi Bruce—do you remember me from undergrad? My name's Laura."

"Of course I remember you, long time no see. You in graduate school now?"

"Yep, it's been a lot of hard work and stress, but in less than a year I'll have my Masters. How's medical school going for you?" *How did she know so much about me? Is there some mutual interest?*

"I feel like I'm finally getting the hang of it," I replied modestly. "It is also pretty challenging and stressful, but after a group of exams, feels oddly rewarding."

"I'll bet . . . where do you live now? Are you on the west side of campus?"

Thus the stage was set for a wondrous two-hour conversation with her, right in the midst of a raucous party. Everything else in the room faded away into a soothing, soft white noise of irrelevance. I was captivated by her joyful energy, her optimism, and interests in people and things. She was beautiful and well-rounded. For the first time since I had gained her acquaintance a few years ago, I believed that we could begin a courtship. Two years later, Laura and I got married and we now have three wonderful daughters. The impact upon my spirit that fall of initial uncertainty was profound. I rediscovered my happiness, and realized that I was deserving of love and respect from others, especially a woman. Subsequently I found myself approaching my existence with a newfound sense of enthusiasm and hopefulness. I remain grateful for the ongoing gifts of her love and support.

As a child my dad took me to many Iowa Hawkeye football games. In the mid-1970s, that really wasn't very exciting. After some fleeting on-field success in the late 1950s, the Hawks hadn't been relevant in the world of college football for nearly twenty years. Classical Big Ten juggernauts such as Michigan and Ohio State would routinely swagger into small Kinnick Stadium and hang 42 points to Iowa mustering a touchdown or two at best. At the time, I was discouraged that my home team was so bereft of any pigskin talent. It was difficult watching the shellacking that our footballers took on a multitude of consecutive fall football Saturdays.

With the passage of time, the disappointment of the on-field losses have eroded away, only to be replaced by a deeper understanding of the nature of competition. When I was a young child, it was easy to become hung up on the scoreboard and the lack of highlights of great plays to display on the gridiron. Though outmatched and outplayed, I admired how my beloved Hawkeyes continued to fight valiantly and press on toward elusive victory, despite the innumerable episodes of being knocked down and intimidated. Sometimes in the arena of life, character isn't found in absolute victory, but rather in the tireless pursuit of accomplishment, getting up off the canvas, and answering the next bell to continue the struggle.

The overwhelming question I have asked myself after coming through incredibly trying experiences is this: When adversity once again lands on my doorstep, what will be my response? Do I naively cower in fear, or attempt to escape my tribulations? I hope to courageously fling open wide the gates, intensely confront my challenges and proclaim, "This is who I am. I am a product of my illustrious heritage, life choices, and both glorious and tragic experiences. Having weathered the storms of grief, fear and depression, I remain unbreakable. My side will carry the days, the months, the years. Despair's abysmal darkness, though seemingly all-encompassing, is fleeting before hope's eternal beacon. This is my ultimate declaration. I stand resolute and unyielding."

It is at that moment that the mantle of manhood will richly hang like a treasured talisman around my tanned and leathered form for all to see. With that internal affirmation, I will have climbed out of my negative valleys, striving for the hilltop of positive self-fulfillment.

CHAPTER 5

LESSONS

Throughout the spectrum of medical training and clinical practice, the common bond which links senior physicians, students, residents and patients together is the concept of education. Like steel sharpening steel, people in the medical world thrive on challenging and learning from each other. Medical students and interns are taught by their senior residents and staff physicians. Health-care professionals of all stripes provide insight, advice and knowledge to patients in hopes of enhancing health and preventing recurrent illness and complications. I have always been surprised by how much I have learned from my patients, whether it is an unusual unanticipated diagnosis, an atypical therapeutic intervention, or even a care situation where I did not perform at my best.

At first glance, the appearance of a dot and a line could not possibly be more divergent in all aspects. A dot is short and definitive, whether it is a period at the end of sentence, capping a short staccato note in a musical composition, or marking a destination on a roadmap. In contrast, a line is long, broad and encompassing or dividing, and can underline a sentence or reading passage for the purpose of emphasis, an answer's blank space on an examination, or to separate lanes on the freeway. In fact, they have been deemed to be so different that Samuel F.B. Morse elected to combine dots and dashes in various combinations when developing and implementing his ubiquitous Morse Code. Unfortunately, a confusion between these two graphic conventions led to a serious medical error and a learning experience during my medical training.

I was an M4, the classification used by the University of Iowa to denote a fourth-year medical student. One of the prestigious rotations as a senior student was serving as a medical subintern for a one-month stint. My assignment was to the Veterans Administration Hospital in Iowa City, a bustling, busy institution with veterans from all wars and backgrounds. It was during this one-month rotation that fourth-years began to assume responsibilities that would be required of them as an intern or resident. The census often was high, workload became significant, and expectations steadily increased over the period of a few weeks.

Early in my rotation, one of my patients was a pleasant gentleman named Max. He was a World War II veteran who had struggled with multiple medical problems, mainly congestive heart failure. He also had a secondary diagnosis of essential thrombocytosis, a condition where the body's bone marrow generates excessive amounts of platelets. High platelets place a patient at increased risk of forming potentially dangerous blood clots. As a result, Max was on a complicated medical regimen, requiring close monitoring of his vital signs, weight, electrolytes and other lab studies. I admitted Max for a congestive heart failure exacerbation, adjusted his medications by increasing his diuretics to decrease his volume load and his digoxin to improve cardiac contractility. He grew stronger, his weight decreased, and his breathing became less labored. After about four days, he was ready to be discharged to home. By that time, the seeds had already been sown for an unfortunate and avoidable medical complication.

The admissions process at the VA was well-established and straightforward. The emergency department would contact the second-year internal medicine resident, who would initially evaluate the patient, complete a brief admission note, write down an updated medication list, and send the patient up to the floor for the first-year intern or fourth-year student to complete the admissions process. In this setting, I would complete my own history and physical examination, write orders and get the patient situated in their hospital room. We would review the medication list that often was hand-copied and written down by our second-year and transcribe it onto the order sheet. On many occasions, the quality of the residents' penmanship presented its own share of risks and pitfalls.

As I perused the list of prescriptions, I noticed an order for Hydrea (hydroxyurea), a medication Max used for his essential thrombocytosis. The dosing of this medication was one of which I was not overly familiar at the time. On the paper, it had the appearance of the following: hydroxyurea 500 mg oral QID (four times per day), which I dutifully copied down on to my order sheet and did not bother to double-check the dosing. In retrospect, maybe I was overly tired or just plain lazy; in any sense, I did not practice due diligence in the review of Max's medications. The actual dose of the Hydrea was actually 500 mg po qd (one time per day). The resident had used capital letters and wrote such a sloppy period, which translated into a line, a letter "I." Thus a qd was bastardized into QID, and a quadrupling of the dose occurred. My fifth grade teacher always warned me that bad penmanship would do me in one day—I just didn't think that it would come about in this fashion.

No immediate impact was noted on his clinical status or lab studies during the remainder of the course of his hospitalization. Four days later, he was discharged without incident to home on his megadose of hydroxyurea, and nothing seemed to be amiss. I forgot about the entire hospitalization until one week later, when I got the call from the ER and the second-year resident—Max was back in the emergency department and was going to need to be rehospitalized, but not for heart failure. On this occasion, my inappropriate megadose of hydroxyurea medication had a devastating effect on all of his blood cell lines, a condition called pancytopenia. His white blood cell count was 1,100/ml (normal 4–10 thousand/ml), hemoglobin (red cell count) was 6.5 gm/dL (normal 13.5–17.0 gm/dL), and platelet count was 45,000/mL (normal 150–400 thousand). By a simple stroke of a pen, I had pulverized the hematopoietic manufacturing plant of his bone marrow into oblivion.

I met Max, apologized to the best of my ability, and who, like many vets, let the adverse situation roll off of his back a little more easily than I thought that he should, given the circumstances. Getting down to business, I readmitted him for the second time in just seven days, and arranged for a couple units of red blood cells and platelets to be transfused over the course of the day due to my carelessness.

Gathering up my things and reorganizing my backpack at the end of the day, I set out for home in the unseasonably warm October late afternoon. I walked with my classmate, Chad Oster, who was doing his subinternship on the other unit at the VA. As I told him of my predicament, I could see his eyes widen, not in self-preservation, but in empathetic fear for my well-being.

"Holy shit, Bruce! You have to present this tomorrow to Martinez at morning report . . . when he finds out what you did, he'll tan your hide!"

"I know . . ." I replied with a mixture of fear and resignation. "I guess I will just have to take my bitter medicine like a man."

Chad and I walked a couple more blocks in silence, then we parted ways toward our respective apartments on the west side of campus. After we exchanged farewell pleasantries, my mood darkened considerably when contemplating having to face Martinez in the morning.

Dr. Martinez was the physician-in-chief for the entire VA hospital internal medicine service. Every Monday through Saturday morning, at 8:00 a.m., all of the services would meet in the large conference room to update the teams on any new admissions and significant changes in condition of any existing patients on the floors. The room was crammed with third-year med students, fourth-year subinterns, first- through third-year residents, fellows, attending physicians, and finally Lord Martinez himself. Dr. Martinez was an incredibly intelligent, well-respected clinician and researcher, accepted absolutely no bullshit, and ate interns alive for breakfast. Any student or resident who was not well-prepared for the morning risked being barked at for lack of thoroughness, interrogated for knowledge deficits, or had their manhood (or womanhood) questioned. That was for seemingly benign and unprovoked clinical offenses. Here I was, with a clear medical error . . . honest mistake it was, but the patient had a significant medically adverse outcome which was my fault, and I bore the lion's share of responsibility for failing the patient when he needed us the most. I had a quick dinner, read up on some of my cases in the internal medicine textbook, then headed off to bed.

For about ninety minutes I laid on my back, restless, and forlornly looked up at the ceiling, feeling awash in a tsunami of self-pity and worry. *What if he yells at me and embarrasses me in front of the entire medical staff? What if I flunk the subinternship and can't graduate in time? What if I get a lousy recommendation for residency from my attending physician?* As my insomnia approached the two-hour mark, and after a few heartfelt prayers to the Almighty, I came upon my answer: No matter how bad it got tomorrow morning, my reply to the Master Inquisitor would go something like this:

Dr. Martinez, I realize that this patient suffered a medical complication solely because of my ineptitude and laziness with regard to medical dosage. What I can tell you is that I admitted my mistake, took immediate steps to correct the problem and make everything right. Finally, I learned a valuable lesson and promise that I will be careful to review med lists and dosages so such a mistake never happens again. At that moment, I realized that he couldn't make me feel any worse about myself and the patient than I was already experiencing. After constructing that short but sweet response in my head, I finally found emotional peace and progressively drifted off to sleep.

The next morning, I reluctantly arose, showered, got dressed and ate my cereal, which felt at the time like my last meal, then made the virtual death march to the VA Hospital. When my time came to give my case summary for my morning report, I stood, cleared the globular lump in my throat, and began a deliberate, a crisp delivery of my case. "Max K. is a pleasant seventy-five-year-old white male, recently seen here and treated for a CHF exacerbation . . ." I continued to outline the series of events, including acknowledging my role in a medical error which resulted in Max's setback and ultimate readmission to the hospital. I also clearly delineated what we had done for our patient since the readmission and explicitly indicated that his condition had stabilized. Dr. Martinez listened with stonefaced thoughtfulness, betraying no sense of emotion. At last he spoke, with a sense of sterility and clinical blandness.

"So his blood counts are better now, and no further complications or new medical issues?"

"Yes, sir," I replied with a slight increased sense of confidence, trying to conceal the fear in my voice and the tremulousness coursing through my legs.

"Fair enough," he concluded matter-of-factly. "Next case." My friend Chad then stood up and began to give the review of his overnight admission.

I couldn't believe it. Here I spent a whole evening worried about the wrath of my attending physician and an accompanying cloud of guilt, shame and incompetence that I was convinced was set to engulf and follow me for all of the days of my professional career. Perhaps what I didn't realize during that day of self-recrimination and remorse, was that I was just as talented and fallible as every other doctor and doctor-to-be in that room. I was able to admit my mistakes, took corrective action, and learned from the experience. In the process, I acknowledged that skill and dedication, along with missteps, in total all compose the colorful palette of the complex world of medicine.

On a cold and rainy October night, Carrie Arenson presented to the labor and delivery floor at Waukesha Memorial Hospital. It was my first month serving as a family medicine resident on the obstetrical service, and I was eager to learn and present a good first impression on the senior obstetricians. Carrie appeared to be in moderate discomfort, huffing and puffing with visible wincing every three to four minutes, the unmistakable signs of active labor. With professional efficiency the nurses got Mrs. Arenson situated into one of the hospital rooms while I reviewed her medical records. Like the majority of the young expectant mothers, she had no major health problems. Her general examination was normal, and her cervical exam showed her to be about 4 cm dilated on the way to complete at 10 cm. The fetal monitor showed contractions every two to three minutes, with the baby's heart rate tolerating the stress of the uterine contractions quite well.

Over the next few hours, Carrie continued to register contractions like clockwork. Around midnight, she felt the urge to push. I checked her cervical exam again immediately. She was completely dilated alright, although the baby was still quite high up in the birth canal, having not descended much.

"Carrie, are you ready to start pushing with the contractions?" I asked.

"Yes, Dr. Rowe, let's get this party going!" she replied. Luckily the epidural anesthetic had relieved most of her pain while not reducing her contractions or ability to hold her legs to push.

"I will let Dr. Dillon know that you are ready, he should be here shortly. In the meantime we can practice pushing along with the contraction."

"OK Doc, sounds good."

Dr. Jack Dillon was a grizzled, established OB/GYN physician who had been in medical practice for thirty years. He had a unrefined demeanor, and the prominent odor of ubiquitous cigarette smoke followed him on his regular morning rounds. He was also capable of great compassion, an excellent surgeon, and one of the smartest clinicians I have ever known.

Within twenty minutes, Dr. Dillon sauntered into Mrs. Arenson's room, and after an exchange of pleasantries, completed a cervical exam of his own. During his check he displayed a quizzical expression. He straightened, removed his gloves and carefully washed his hands.

"OK, just so you know, Carrie, your baby is coming down face-side up, not down. That means that your labor is going to be at least a couple more hours before this baby comes. I am going to hang out in the call room for now, and Dr. Rowe will help you with the pushing. Good luck and keep me posted."

"Thanks Dr. Dillon," Carrie and I replied almost in unison, both of us disappointed that we still had a fair amount of work in front of us.

I felt some righteous indignation toward Dr. Dillon that night, especially since I was new, didn't know him very well, and was bereft of any significant obstetrical experience. *Two more hours of labor, huh? I'll show that sonofabitch that with some hard work we'll get this baby out in no time. In fact, we might go so fast that he'll end up missing the whole thing!*

Every three minutes, Carrie and her husband, the nurse and I would re-enact the classic delivery passion play: contraction coming, deep breath in, push for three sets of ten seconds, then relax, and repeat three minutes later. Soon fifteen minutes of effort became thirty, then sixty, then nearly two hours flew by. We were all rapidly approaching resignation when almost on cue Dr. Dillon made an encore appearance.

"Hey guys, are were making any progress yet?" too nonchalantly and overconfident for my taste.

"We've really been trying hard," I replied with obvious resignation. "But unfortunately it has been slow going." *Maybe she's going to need a C-section.*

"Well, let's have another look here, shall we?" Dr. Dillon cheerfully inquired and repeated the cervical check. "The baby has come down somewhat and now the face is pointing sideways, so I think something is going to happen soon. When your next contraction comes, I want you to push down hard against my fingers, understand?" He was now in his element, politely confident and focused on the patient and the job at hand.

"OK Doctor," Carrie replied with more than a hint of exhaustion.

Three minutes later the wave of uterine muscular expulsion arrived. As Carrie pushed down, Dr. Dillon used his fingers in the birth canal to gently coax to baby's head to rotate into a facedown position. He almost got it on the first try. The second attempt three minutes later was successful; the fontanel indicated that things had moved into the right place.

Once the baby's head was oriented facedown, the impact was dramatic. The vertex of the baby's scalp came forward immediately to the vaginal opening, and after one more set of pushes little Jacob was born.

"Congrats guys . . . he's a cutie," Dr. Dillon proclaimed. "Bruce, can you stitch the small abrasion there? I'm going home to catch some shut-eye."

"OK sure, Dr. Dillon, thanks." Just like that, he vanished into the night. There was no gloating, grand teaching gesture or prolonged interaction. The successful work of a flawless, beautiful delivery laid bare for all to see, and it spoke for itself. I learned to respect the gift of experience and appreciate the aura of confidence that my senior physicians could offer me, even if I didn't always like the package it came in.

My third-year medical school general internal medicine clerkship took place at the University Hospital in Iowa City. While some of my classmates dreaded the peculiarities of the patients with their complex medical problems, social issues and psychiatric maladies, I embraced the setting. The sights, smells and bustling activity on the floors was exciting and stimulating, making every day an unpredictable crapshoot.

About two weeks in to my six-week rotation, Mr. Keeney presented to our service. He had a complicated medical history, including COPD, congestive heart failure, and osteoarthritis. On this admission, his presenting complaint was more atypical and unusual—he had a severe, unrelenting sensation of itching, called pruritus, for several weeks that was progressively worsening. His itching persisted everywhere, and the skin all over his body, including arms, legs and trunk, was covered with substantial papules, excoriations and scratch marks. He arrived on the floor brandishing a very stiff and barbaric-appearing toilet bowl brush that he utilized to scratch his back whenever it was deemed necessary. From the initial introductions and subsequent examination, the entire global aspect of the case just seemed weird, and when I began to interview Mr. Keeney and his wife, things became even more awkward.

Mrs. Keeney began first. "I'm tellin' you, it's from that water pill, Lasix, that he's been on for the last few months. Maybe we should just stop it."

As a relatively fresh third-year medical student, I felt compelled to flex my intellectual muscles and hold my ground in this case. *How can this layperson know anything about clinical pharmacology and medicinal side effects?* It was a pretty arrogant attitude in retrospect, but when a young, insecure doctor is trying to establish his control of the situation and projecting self-confidence, this is frequently the result. "I have never heard of such a side effect from Lasix like this previously. Plus, if we stop this medication for him, he will retain fluid and go into heart failure again."

The Keeneys seemed nonplussed by my initial assessment of the role of medications. "Are you sure, Doc?" asked Mr. Keeney tactfully. "This itching is drivin' me crazy, I can't even sleep at night at this point."

"We've washed all of the bedding, changed soaps and laundry detergents, and nothing is helping. I've been givin' him Benadryl like candy, and it's not touching it," piped Mrs. Keeney.

I reviewed the medication list, but nothing jumped out at me that would cause pruritus. Niacin and opioid pain medications are examples of some of the big offenders—he was on neither. He had not used any unusual lotions, detergents or perfumes recently, and no new fabrics or unusual travel history noted. Carefully, I began to construct a differential diagnosis in my mind. *Atopic or contact dermatitis? Bedbug infestation or scabies? Autosensitization dermatitis? Psychogenic sensation of itchiness?* I was beginning to gravitate toward the latter, given the lack of supporting evidence from the patient's history and physical examination. In the interim, I tried treating him with multiple antihistamines, including hydroxyzine, but that only made him tired, and he continued to scratch madly at himself. I contemplated using an oral corticosteroid such as prednisone to treat his rash, but hesitated because I did not have an accurate diagnosis yet.

A couple of days went by, the family became increasingly exasperated, and I remained intransigent in my belief that it was some obscure and idiopathic cause, not related to any of his current medications. Mrs. Keeney buttonholed me in the hallway after I had completed my morning rounds. She understandably projected frustration and irritation while advocating simultaneously for her husband.

"Listen Doc, you gotta help my Donnie and get this deal figured out. Either find the right answer and medication for him or get rid of the stupid Lasix, OK?" She sounded insistent and righteously indignant. In my juvenile mind it was a perceived doctor vs. patient battle, not a partnership between family and physician to get to the root of the problem. It sure seemed to me that the Keeneys had the upper hand now. I reassured her that I would review the case with my attending that afternoon, and we would have a treatment plan by the end of the day. At that juncture, I toyed with the idea of calling in a dermatology consult, but they often didn't like coming into the hospital, and I wasn't ready to admit diagnostic defeat.

With a bit of an attitude and misplaced sense of self-righteousness, I discussed Mr. Keeney's issues with my attending about an hour later. "The family is convinced that the itching is due to the Lasix, but I fail to see the connection."

My attending was not moved by my assessment. "Did you hold the Lasix for a couple of days just to see what happens?"

"No—I didn't think it would be worthwhile. I don't see how Lasix would cause that severe of a pruritus and a rash. Plus he might begin to retain fluid."

"C'mon now, let's humor the family and see what happens here. You know that we can closely monitor his body weight and fluid status here in the hospital, and if it's psychogenic, the power of suggestion may also help with his itching as well."

Chastened by my attending's suggestion, I took her advice and discontinued his Lasix. Over the next few days, the pruritus abated, the excoriations and rash improved, and the toilet brush was relegated back to a bathroom usage only. Mr. Keeney and his wife were delighted. They thanked me for my care during their hospitalization, but in actuality I should have been expressing my gratitude to them for their insights and patient advocacy. In my reading later that week, I came upon the realization that Lasix has sulfhydryl compounds in its chemical structure. A nontrivial subset of patients have sulfa allergies of varying degrees of intensity. Most likely, Mr. Keeney had a dermatological manifestation of a sulfa-type allergy. The Keeneys ultimately had been correct about the situation all along.

From that point forward, with respect to medication and side effects, I developed the following five-part mantra, The Rule of Any:

Any medication
Can cause *any* side effect
For *any* person
At *any* time
For *any* reason

It has served me well with countless patient interactions since that initial powerful, humbling clinical experience. It affirms the concerns that the patient may have about a medication side effect, and compels me to dig deeper in a patient's medication list. In the process, I may learn about a new obscure medication side effect, or provide reassurance to a patient that the medication does not appear to be the culprit.

Through the years, I have always been grateful for the lessons that my patients have so generously taught me. Whether an unusual case, strange family dynamics, obscure therapeutic interventions, or a personal opportunity for clinical improvement, there exists the humbling realization that as a physician, my educational journey will never be complete. As I pass the seeds of my medical knowledge and experiences to the upcoming generations of medical professionals, I hope that the refinement of the educational bonds between doctors, students and patients will enrich us all.

CHAPTER 6

MISMATCH

My late father had many unique sayings and pearls of advice, some of which he repetitively drilled into my consciousness. One of my favorites was, "Bruce, find your niche, locate your place in this world where you'll be happy and succeed." I have reflected on that intellectual nugget during times when I have struggled to find my role in the grand scheme of life.

In the growing hours of darkness and chilliness of late October, my eighth grade football season had mercifully come to a close. I trudged home following our last game, a 35–7 drubbing at the hands of a much-hated and athletically superior neighboring town. My lone contribution was a three-yard carry as a fourth-string tailback in the supplemental extra time after the game, known as the Fifth Quarter. During that short block of bonus fluff time, all of the scrubs including myself got a chance, albeit meaningless, to receive some in-game action. At the end of my single rushing attempt, any temporary satisfaction with my short gain was quashed by an awful gang tackle. I heard the obnoxious grunts and felt the incredible crushing weight of multiple defenders inappropriately piling upon me well after the referee's whistle. I hobbled to my feet, finally free of the oppressive, heavy conglomeration of extremities and bodies. Shaken, I looked to the referee, hoping that a yellow penalty flag had been thrown for unnecessary roughness. Our eyes met, and the official walked over to me. However, all he said was, "Hey buddy, if that happened in the actual game, we would have called a penalty."

Oh that's just great! Thanks for looking out for my safety, well-being and a clean game . . .

On my ten-minute walk home after the ignominious defeat, every muscle in my undersized body ached, each respectively crying out for my attention. Simple activities like turning and breathing became challenging, requiring an unreasonable level of effort. I felt discouraged, contemplating the futile exercise throughout middle school of trying to be a decent football player. Like all of my fellow aspiring athletes, I wanted to become strong and popular, respected by boys and coveted by the girls.

Although I enjoyed watching football live and on television, I had grown to detest participating in the game itself. I hated the incessant drilling, being yelled at by the coaching staff, spending countless hours in the baking sun and brutal cold. Practicing for an activity where I lacked skills and had minimal opportunity for meaningful athletic impact was losing its luster. Bigger and stronger teammates would target me to be on the receiving end of the most vicious tackles and occasional cheap shots. It was clear that my heart was no longer into playing football. As I despondently stepped over the threshold into my house, I steeled myself for the disappointment from my father regarding this decision and prepared myself for a battle of wills.

My parents had made it home before me, and my father noticed my tentative entrance into the door. "Hey man, pretty tough game out there today, huh?"

"Yeah, for just playing during the junk time of the game, the other team still felt compelled to dish out a lot of hits and tackles," I replied dejectedly. "So they wiped the floor with us and I got clobbered."

"Way to hang in there and try to help your team," my mother countered, in a mighty attempt to project positivity.

"I guess so . . . Hey listen . . . Mom, Dad, I've given it a lot of thought, and I've decided to quit playing football for our school after this year. I'm not that talented, and frankly I don't enjoy playing the sport much at all for a variety of reasons. Hope you guys aren't too mad at me . . ."

Following this unexpected drop of surprising news, there was a protracted silence, on the cusp of being uncomfortable. My dad took off his reading glasses, looked up from the daily newspaper and eyed me with a combination of concern and suspicion.

"Are you sure that this is what you want to do?" he queried, with awkward uncertainty.

"Yes, Dad—I don't see any prospects of me getting better, and even if I did improve, I still wouldn't enjoy it. Sorry to disappoint you . . ."

My dad's eyes narrowed, accompanied by a subtle furrowing of his eyebrows. I couldn't tell at first if he was angry or worried about my well-being. I prepped myself for a barrage of questions about my level of commitment and manhood, and him building his case for investing another year in the gridiron trenches. Interestingly, his demeanor did not project hostility or frustration. Rather, he was suppressing a smile, and when he spoke he sounded genuinely curious about my future plans.

"Is this what you really want to do, Bruce?" he asked again, now with an increased tone of seriousness.

"Yes Dad, I guess I'm just not cut out for this jock stuff, maybe I should just stick to the band, choir and the plays . . ."

"Bruce, how many different sports teams and athletic clubs are there in the high school?"

"I dunno, maybe about twelve to fifteen, I guess."

"Who told you that the only path to athletic excellence is through the three sports that you have tried so far? Be brave and attempt new things, push past your comfort zone, find your sporting niche. I believe there's an athletic activity in your school where you can succeed."

"OK Dad, thanks for that advice, I appreciate that."

Even though at that moment I felt completely beaten down and defeated, those inspiring words fanned a flickering flame of courage. Instead of sensing the drumbeat of trepidation regarding an upcoming sports season, I embraced the optimism of possibilities. The following fall, my shoulder pads and cleats were supplanted by running shoes and a singlet as my uniform, and I never looked back—I had finally found my sporting niche! Four years later, as a six-time letter winner in cross country and track, I discovered that I could excel in athletics on my own terms.

It was late summer in Iowa City, and I was immersed in the second rotation of my third year of medical school, a six-week stint on the obstetrics and gynecology service. After completing the first half of the program on the labor and delivery unit, I was now assigned to the outpatient gynecology clinic.

My third patient of the morning was a nice middle-aged African American woman named Phyllis. She presented with some heavy irregular bleeding, cramping and passage of blood clots. Upon pelvic examination I noted that she had an enlarged, irregular uterus related to multiple benign fibroid tumors. At some point she was going to need a hysterectomy. While listening to her heart and lungs, however, I heard a fair amount of wheezing scattered throughout all of her lung fields.

"Phyllis, do you have a history of asthma?"

"Why yes I do, do my lungs sound bad today?"

"Yes, I hear a lot of wheezing all over your chest. Do you normally take inhalers for your breathing issues?"

"Yes, but I ran out of them several months ago. I guess I was busy and I never got around to calling my doctor for my refills."

"I'll tell you what. I can talk with my attending, and at the end of your visit I can give you a prescription refill on your inhalers. You can pick them up at the pharmacy later today."

"That would be lovely, thanks so much, kind young doctor."

Happily, I left the room and went to present my case to my senior chief resident. Brent Miller had the reputation for being an intelligent and technically skilled OB/GYN physician. Unfortunately, his well-known and established penchant for being a complete asshole also preceded him. I spent a few minutes describing Phyllis's story: her enlarged fibroid uterus, plan for a pelvic ultrasound and a follow-up gynecologic surgical consultation, to which he heartily agreed. I then brought up the concern I had with my patient's wheezing.

"I also happened to check out her lungs today, and she sounds very wheezy. She has chronic asthma. I think we should renew the prescription for her inhal—"

Dr. Miller, in his classic undiplomatic manner, interrupted me with his harsh rhetoric. "What the hell, Bruce? This is an OB/GYN clinic, not a primary care clinic. We don't have time to deal with all of these little side issues. You will *not* refill any inhalers for her today. Refer her back to the pulmonary or internal medicine clinic, for Christ's sake!" He gave me a dismissive look and turned back to some paperwork on his desk, terminating our conversation.

With a thick air of resignation, I turned on my heels and wordlessly departed the office. A few minutes later, I communicated my treatment plan to Phyllis, giving a flimsy reason for not refilling her inhaler prescription. She expressed some mild disappointment but also understood the peculiar process of a tertiary care hospital. As instructed, I gave her a referral to the internal medicine clinic and wished her well. I never heard from her again, but I hoped that she had both her pulmonary and gynecologic problems resolved.

At the conclusion of that visit, I felt a double dose of discouragement, between Phyllis sensing my clinical inadequacy and my narrow-minded chief resident handcuffing my desire to practice comprehensive patient medical care. I started to realize that I may not be an ideal fit for an academic institution to practice medicine after completing my medical training. Tertiary and academic medical centers thrive on focused, specialized medical care, and that is important and useful. However, I am a big-picture type of clinician, and I enjoy taking care of people, not organ systems. It was becoming clear that my skill set and interests would match up better in a primary care-type clinical setting. Unfortunately, in a large Big Ten university, anchored by a high-powered medical school, teaching hospital and research institution environment, I was uncertain if this was the best use of my talents. Sizable numbers of my classmates were heading toward prestigious, glamorous specialties, and I could hold my own with the vast majority of them. I found myself struggling with my future choice of specialty; do I use my medical talents to pursue a high-powered, stressful residency in the competitive arena of orthopaedic surgery, or acknowledge my personality and interests, and gravitate toward a primary care field? The next chapter of my life's ever-changing saga was rapidly unfolding, and I hoped that I was ready for whatever crazy circumstances the future had in store.

The first year of medical school is one of the most stimulating and stressful experiences of a young graduate's life, and it was especially so for me. Losing my father eight months before starting medical school cast a pall over a normally exciting life adventure. I debated taking a gap year, but ultimately decided I needed to keep moving forward, with my best friend Jason. I missed my dad terribly, felt guilty about leaving my mom and sister alone at home to fend for themselves, and I had lost some of my motivation and dedication.

Initially I struggled with the coursework due to the shadow of grief affecting my concentration, as opposed to any academic deficit. Attempting to digest an overwhelming quantity of material, spending countless hours studying, working with equally driven and intelligent classmates was a significant challenge. The pungent smell of formaldehyde from the gross anatomy lab permeated my clothes in those early training days, leading to some strange looks by my fellow riders on the morning campus bus ride. One night, getting ready for bed, I was horrified to find a piece of my cadaver's fatty tissue wedged behind my belt buckle. I completed the last of my spring freshman final examinations, straining to keep my eyes open and hold my head upright due to sheer exhaustion. Despite the nagging sense of loss and occasional crises of self-confidence, I felt blessed getting through that harrowing first year.

The final year of medical school in contrast is sometimes more like a victory lap. Students can utilize their interests to custom design any curriculum. Rotations were more focused and enjoyable. As late fall and winter approached, students headed out on the interview circuit to rub elbows with faculty and directors of the residency programs. After finding out their residency destination in March, most students could coast along until the May graduation ceremony.

Almost imperceptibly, my reality began to slowly deviate from my mental fourth-year fairy tale. I had decided on orthopedic surgery as my specialty, but learned early on in the postgraduate residency selection process that I had chosen one of the most competitive specialties. Orthopedic surgery applicants had incredible intellect and compelling life stories. Many of the students had research already published, were NCAA Division

I athletes, and were graduating near or at the very top of their respective medical school classes. There was going to be a brutal competition for the five hundred orthopedic residency slots available nationwide. My academic and life adventures were less memorable, and my journey on the interview trail quickly became intimidating.

After submitting applications to sixty-two orthopedic residency programs, I was only accepted for an interview at seventeen of them. In three consecutive days in December, I drove from Pittsburgh to Columbus, Ohio to Indianapolis, an exhausting itinerary. The questions I fielded from various residency faculty ranged from the obtuse (What are your opinions on cheating?), the annoying (Why aren't you at the very top of your class?), to the irrelevant (What three famous people would you invite to dinner?). Despite the incredibly discouraging process, I held out hope that my well-above-average academic performance and strong letters of recommendation would help me to succeed.

During the last semester of our medical school career, in late March, comes the special date that all medical students excitedly look forward to for three and a half-plus years: Match Day. On this momentous occasion, the entire fourth-year class gathers in the commons area and opens up a small envelope. Inside are the all-important contents, which reveal to the impending medical school graduate their practice specialty and training location. Much like a fraternity or sorority rush, students and residency programs rank each other, and where both of the preferences line up the highest is where a young physician will be placed. Though often a stressful selection, for most students is a joyous occasion, the crowning achievement of a long educational effort.

About 70 percent of the students get their first pick of residency program, and usually 90 percent get one of their top three choices. As the weeks leading up to the Match approached, I felt a mixture of excitement and apprehension. Finding out what resided within that envelope became an all-consuming preoccupation.

Two days prior to the official Match Day, on a Monday afternoon, the graduating seniors met in the auditorium and received another plain white envelope with their name written on it. Inside was a brief note indicating simply whether you successfully matched to a residency position. The final destination was listed in the envelope on the Match Day ceremony two days later. Nervously, I awaited my simple yet powerful envelope. Having an "R" surname always required an inordinate level of patience.

At last I received my boarding pass to the next stage of my career. I quietly walked down to an abandoned corridor, and with trembling hands awkwardly tore open the envelope. As I begin to read, the soul-crushing news spilled out on the page, the barren Times New Roman sentence of disappointment, one awful word at a time:

We regret to inform you that you have not successfully matched to a residency position for this upcoming year.

I couldn't believe it . . . all of the hard work, great letters of recommendation, solid grades academically, after getting past my grief for my dad . . . and for what? Rejection crashed through at a point that was supposed to be one of the high-water marks of my life. A treasured position I believed that I richly deserved had inexplicably slipped out of my grasp. Never in my life had I failed so completely and spectacularly at something that I had so desperately wanted. Instead of being filled with pride and happiness, Match Day for me would now be a public embarrassment. What was I going to say to my fiancée Laura and my medical school roommate Jason? *What was the point of willing my body, mind and spirit that freshman fall term of medical school and every challenging succeeding semester, shrouded in sadness and despair only months after my dad died, to complete a special quest . . . was this how my dream was supposed to turn out? Why didn't anyone like me? What did I say or do on my interviews that derailed my future plans?*

Trying to be inconspicuous as possible, I quickly exited out of a side door for home. I walked briskly, head bowed, a mixture of profound disappointment and sheer anger. The late afternoon March sun remained too low in the sky, and a harsh stinging wind cruelly knifed through the still-leafless trees. Sadly, I called Laura and gave her the bad news, followed by copious mutual tears.

Unfortunately, there was no time for self-reflection—we needed to prepare for the next morning, referred to as Tuesday Scramble Day. Over several stressful hours, all of the remaining unmatched medical students frantically called around the country to find a position to begin their residency training. Laura was already finishing a speech pathology Clinical Fellowship Year out in Philadelphia, so we decided that I should search for a transitional internship out East. By 11:00 a.m. on Tuesday, I had committed to Presbyterian Hospital in Philadelphia for a single year of internship studies. Although I remained disappointed, I was relieved to have secured a residency position.

Match Day officially arrived on Wednesday, when everyone else found out their actual residency assignments. It was an incredibly tough morning: Every opened envelope, smile and joyous scream from my successfully chosen classmates felt like a dispiriting blow to my fragile ego. For weeks I woke up every morning, futilely hoping that the entire fiasco was just an awful nightmare. As much as I wished for things to have turned out differently, I needed to quickly pick up the pieces and move positively forward with my life.

Several weeks after Match Day, the final spring semester drew to a close, followed by medical school graduation. As we recited the Hippocratic Oath and I received my dark-green graduate Doctor of Medicine hood, I felt humbled and privileged to finally be joining the honorable fraternity of medicine. I lightly tapped my right front pants pocket. Within it was a buckeye that I found in Laura's backyard home in southeastern Iowa, my late dad's traditional good luck charm. As I crossed the stage, I glanced skyward at end of my journey. *We did it, Dad!* Although the initial residency plans had disastrously collapsed, the precious physician dream was realized.

After graduation, I allowed my optimism and excitement about the next stage of training reenter my soul. Laura and I married a month later, and we loaded up a small moving truck and brought all of my worldly possessions out East to suburban Philly. Within days I was working very long and challenging hours as a surgical intern in a bustling, urban hospital.

Immersion in a challenging general surgical rotation during my transitional internship was the perfect salve to the residual shame and disappointment I harbored about the orthopedic residency mismatch. I didn't possess the time or mental energy to dwell on the perceived slights and shortcomings of the past. I needed to place the unpleasant experience behind me and keep moving forward in my clinical training. As my internship year progressed, like steel hardened in fire, I began to grow in confidence in my abilities. I realized that I displayed good technical skills in the OR, compassionately related to my patients, and developed a knack for juggling many complicated patients and situations. After several challenging months, I sensed my progressive growth as a young healer.

I earnestly believe that my personal setbacks took place with a greater sense of purpose in mind. Sometimes it is difficult for me to see the big picture, and I get lost in the immediate problem while neglecting my long-term life arc. Several months into my internship year, this was illustrated in jarring fashion. I had carved out a few free moments in the hospital library to read the *Philadelphia Inquirer.* Frequently I would peruse the obituary pages to see if any of our clinic patients had recently passed away. Midway down the first page, a tragic death notice dramatically caught my attention.

"Dr. Anthony Gennaro, a highly regarded orthopaedic surgeon, died suddenly and unexpectedly of a heart attack at age 46. He is survived by his loving wife, Melinda, as well as a son and two daughters. Dr. Gennaro was a highly respected surgeon and the author of multiple research publications and book chapters . . ."

Was this God attempting to send me a message? I could have embarked on a prestigious medical track, with prospects for renown and accolades. It cannot be stated with certainty that job stress directly produced Dr. Gennaro's tragic circumstances. However, I realized that with *my* family history of cardiac disease, the stress of a challenging orthopedic surgery lifestyle could wear me down and destroy me in the prime of middle age. A few weeks later, I made the momentous decision to apply for a family medicine residency closer to home in the Upper Midwest for the following academic year. My wife was relieved that I was pursuing something that for me was a better speciality match.

In midwinter, as I embarked on a second annual course of residency interviews, the previously agonizing tenor of the process was now completely different. Everyone seemed interested in me as a person and my backstory, and eager to bring me in as a new resident physician. Laura and I opted to move to suburban Milwaukee so I could take on a second-year family medicine position. Children's Hospital of Wisconsin hired Laura to work as a pediatric speech pathologist. Twenty years later, we continue to make our home here in America's Dairyland with our three daughters. Frequently an unanticipated deviation from my life's expected path is often not just a painful detour; rather, it may open up a previously unknown new skill set, opportunity or passion.

Lauren Allen was a thirty-seven-year-old, delightful, recently remarried mother of two rambunctious sons. She had been healthy except for some issues with mild elevations in blood pressure and cholesterol. One day we squeezed her in for an urgent care appointment because of some persistent abdominal pain. Normally, Lauren had a gregarious and engaging personality. However, something seemed a little bit off during her appointment. She was visibly uncomfortable, and appeared to be haggard and sleep deprived. A sheaf of papers from a visit to our local tertiary care center emergency department last evening accompanied her. She had a thorough examination there, along with a complete battery of lab tests and an abdominal ultrasound, all of which were unremarkable.

I tried to maintain some level of cheer while being considerate of her medical predicament. "Hi Lauren, sounds like you had a rough night."

"Yeah Doc, my sleeping could've been a lot better, that's for sure. This pain's been horrible lately, especially overnight."

"Can you show me where the pain is located?"

"Right here." She gestured toward her right upper quadrant region of the abdomen. That is typically an area where liver and gallbladder problems originate.

"How bad's the pain been, on a scale from 1 to 10?"

She didn't hesitate in her response. "About a 7 or an 8 most days, it's been really bad the last few weeks."

"Is it a sharp pain, or a dull ache? Does it move around anywhere?"

"Mostly dull ache, sometimes sharp at night. Doesn't really move around much."

"Do you have a lot of gas and bloating symptoms?"

"Yes . . . a lot!"

"Is it worse after eating fatty foods?"

"I don't know, it seems to be pretty bad all of the time right now."

I reviewed her lab results and negative abdominal ultrasound report from the ER, including the finding of a normal-appearing gallbladder. On physical exam, Lauren had a fair amount of abdominal pain over the right upper quadrant region. She also displayed a positive Murphy's sign, in which a patient interrupts a deep inspiration with an examiner's deep pressure over the gallbladder. She had no indications of diffuse severe abdominal tenderness, which would indicate a surgical emergency.

I was a little perplexed at this point. "Lauren," I asked, "what did the ER staff believe was the cause of your abdominal pain?"

"I don't know, it was kinda weird. They said all of my tests were normal, so it most likely was reflux disease. So they gave me some kind of stomach medicine and sent me home."

Upon reviewing her case in its entirety, clearly there was an incongruence, a mismatch between Lauren's clinical presentation and her test results. Despite her results being "normal," she had all of the clinical indications that one would expect in a setting of acute gallbladder disease, also known as cholecystitis/biliary colic. I contemplated an internal mantra I use to help guide me in clinical dilemmas:

Treat the patient, not the lab results.
What is the patient trying to tell you?

I knew that I had to downplay the so-called normal test results and continue to work up Lauren's problem as if she was suffering from an inflamed gallbladder. Was there any other lab study or test that could help me out of this quandary? Why, of course! We could check a HIDA scan, a nuclear medicine test that examines the physiology of the gallbladder, specifically whether it fills and empties appropriately. I arranged for the HIDA scan to be completed later that afternoon, and not surprisingly, the gallbladder was not functioning properly. Two days later, her gallbladder was removed, and showed both inflammation and a large gallstone lodged high in the neck of the gallbladder, which explained why it was not visualized on her ultrasound exam. Lauren made a full recovery; her situation is a reminder that the primary objective is to heal and comfort patients, and not treat inanimate pieces of paper.

Whether on the unforgiving football field, a difficult residency discernment, or a patient with discordant diagnostic clues, the concept of fitting in and matching up in life's settings is often challenging. Through the years, I have needed to balance my internal self-confidence with my external talents and opportunities. I have cultivated my medical gifts while also making the difficult acknowledgement that certain abilities for me will continue to remain elusive. In my profession I have made it a priority to not permit modern medical technology to override my discussions of patient's history and their physical exam findings. Navigating these weighty issues has allowed me to settle in a niche where I feel a sense of spiritual contentment and belonging.

CHAPTER 7

TRANSFORM

It was a warm late-summer day, and the year had been one of mixed blessings. The joy of welcoming a new niece into the family was tempered by the sudden passing of Laura's grandfather Len. He was the quintessential gregarious South Side of Chicago Polish patriarch: seven children, usher in the local Catholic church, worked in the produce section of the Jewel grocery store for forty-plus years. He loved spending spring and summer working in his backyard, replete with a lovingly tended flower garden and a myriad of birds and butterflies. A heart attack on an early May afternoon claimed him abruptly in the living room of his home. For weeks after his funeral, members of the extended family began to report sightings of monarch butterflies in the yards around their homes. What began as a few anecdotes became multiple stories of increasing frequency and detail. Initially, I approached the stories with a degree of skepticism; maybe our family was subconsciously attempting to achieve a spiritual connection with Len.

I set about the weekly ritual of mowing my yard on a bright August afternoon. Halfway through my lawn manicuring a solitary monarch butterfly made a dramatic appearance and playfully danced around my head, as if to say, "It's me, Papa, I'm OK in heaven, everything's great here." Subliminally, I felt a profound sense of peace and love, grateful for a perceived outward sign of an afterlife.

Two weeks later, an additional blessing revealed itself in our garden: on our milkweed plants, ten black-and-gold striated monarch butterfly caterpillars, voraciously devouring the vegetation. Over the succeeding days I witnessed the caterpillars steadily grow and molt. Finally, the ultimate incredible transfiguration—a turquoise, golden-dotted chrysalis, followed by the emergence of a spectacular butterfly ten days later. I humbly realized that out of a dark and oppressive life space, a beautiful resurrection can be manifest.

"Oh crap . . . This is really complicated . . ." I thought dejectedly, staring at the seemingly incomprehensible worksheet of mathematical problems. As a sophomore biomedical engineering major, I was not spending a lovely October Saturday outside for a run or listening to a Hawkeye football away game on the radio. Instead, I was holed up in the engineering library, trying to wrestle with a bewildering array of homework assignments.

With a disappointed, wistful glance I stared out of the classic, large warped windowpanes onto the Pentacrest, the central park space hub of the University of Iowa campus and home of the iconic Old Capitol building. Many of the oak, maple and chestnut trees were rapidly approaching peak color with brilliant warm autumnal hues. An ongoing gentle sprinkling of scarlet, golden and orange leaves cascaded onto the barren sidewalks below the trees' graceful upward-arching branches. Days like these made me question why I chose a challenging major like engineering in combination with the demands of the premedical track. *Shouldn't I just decide on one or the other, and not try to do both?* I fought the distracting temptations and reluctantly pressed on while many of my fellow students strolled the campus and basked in the cool, slanted sunlight under the chromatic canopy.

My current class nemesis was titled *Intro to Differential Equations*, a higher-level mathematical course that many engineering students dreaded, simply referring to the class as "Diffy Q." So far I had sailed through my calculus and lower-level mathematics classes with relative ease. Diffy Q was proving to be a humbling and stern taskmaster, and I was struggling with even the most basic concepts. Despite the encouragement from my professor, a bookish angular Dane named Dr. Pedersen, I could only muster a low "B" on the first midterm exam. I feared that I was in over my head and worried, as this class was a prerequisite for upper-level engineering courses.

As I sat wrestling with the page of intimidating calculations, a kind acquaintance named Julian pulled up a chair to chat. Julian was also a sophomore and had survived Diffy Q last spring.

"Hi ya, Bruce—how's it goin'? Didn't think I'd see you inside doing homework on a lovely fall Saturday afternoon such as this. I'm only here because I have a design project due on Monday," he quipped cheerfully. Julian worked hard, so it wasn't surprising that he would sacrifice a fantastic autumn day to try and get ahead. Still, all of the engineering stuff came a little bit more naturally to him. "Hmmm . . . Diffy Q, huh? Are you gettin' it figured out?"

I stared blankly at him for a few awkward moments, then answered with a surprisingly weary voice, "As a matter of fact, no, I don't understand this at all. I did great in all of my math courses up until now."

My lamentations did not unnerve Julian in the least. "Now c'mon, Bruce, you're a smart guy; think it through, and you can always use a Laplace transform to make your work easier, that was my saving grace in that class . . ."

Laplace transform? We were just starting to learn about that concept. In the mathematical and engineering realm, a Laplace transform takes a complicated mathematical function, changes it into a more simplistic one, and after an appropriate calculation, can be changed back into a similarly complicated end result. It is magical that you can work with the variables and operations more easily in that format. Julian sat down beside me and we worked through a few of the problems. I steadily grew in confidence and displayed a newfound proficiency with the calculations.

Gratefully, I thanked Julian for his insights and set off for home in the hopes of getting outside for the last fading vestiges of the daylight. Fortunately, I carried that intellectual momentum forward with me to salvage an "A" for the course. I appreciated the power that day of the Laplace transform, not only to impact a problem set on paper, but also upon my academic journey. With each succeeding semester, I became convinced that I could not only tackle the problems posed in the engineering world, but also the intellectual complexities of medicine.

During the winter term of our sophomore year of high school, every student was required to take a ballroom dancing unit for gym class. Without exception, it was detested by every male in the student body. Every boy was paired with a socially awkward girl, and they were forced to dance together for an entire class period. Furthermore, the head football coach was our teacher, and every guy had to hit a middle-ground sweet spot in his approach to dancing style: perform too lackadaisically and you could encounter the ire of the head coach and a bad grade, while too much enthusiasm resulted in derision and ridicule from your fellow male classmates.

On our first day, we reluctantly hit the ground running with our dance partners after our teacher stated in no uncertain terms that poor attitudes and lack of effort would not be tolerated. Over a period of several weeks, we perfected waltzes, swing dances, jitterbugs, polkas, cha-chas, tangos, and square dances. Begrudgingly, every student made steady improvement with executing the different styles of the most common ballroom dances. At the conclusion of this protracted unit, we were relieved to put the course of events behind us and embraced a competitive unit on basketball.

I never gave the class a second thought until several years later. During the summer months approaching my senior year of college, there were several weddings for my high school and college classmates. Invariably, at every wedding was a reception, complete with a disc jockey and a plethora of dancing. With relative ease, my buddies and I recalled the styles and movements of all of the ballroom dances. Confidently, I asked many girls to join me on the floor for a waltz, polka or jitterbug. Almost universally they acquiesced, and we both enjoyed stepping and turning to the joyous music. Quietly under my breath I thanked my high school football coach for pushing me to perfect my dance skills. It was a surprising blessing and revelation for me to enjoy the interest and company of the now-pretty girls, who were metamorphosing into alluring and beautiful young women.

Early in my second year of medical school, I met my lovely wife Laura, and during our courtship we attended her cousin's wedding together. Of course, it was a large Roman Catholic Polish ceremony held on South Side of Chicago. Later in the evening, during the reception, a happy and jaunty accordion lead-in blared over the speakers—I immediately knew which ballroom dance was coming up next.

"Do you know how to polka?" Laura inquired innocently.

Out of the corner of my vision, I caught a glimpse of my future father-in-law, Jim. Our eyes met, and he appeared to give me a slight wink. His demeanor was partial encouragement coupled with curiosity about my next move.

"Yeah, I've done it a few times," I replied nonchalantly.

Laura and I strode out onto the dance floor with the excited, clapping mass of humanity. I could subconsciously sense many adjacent eyes trained upon me, sizing me up in terms of my polkaing prowess. As we effortlessly synchronized our hopping, joyful moves across the brown parquet surface, I began to feel grateful for the transformative experience of dance. It was a simple polka, but doing it well allowed a small-town, Protestant Iowa boy to find his way into the hearts of a welcoming Chicago Polish Catholic family.

During my third year medical school clerkships, I was assigned to an internal medicine subspecialty service for a three-week rotation. I had requested cardiology, thinking it would be exciting and expose me to the high-profile, challenging world of heart disease. Instead, to my disappointment and chagrin I found myself on the hematology-oncology service. My initial impressions of "heme-onc" were that of dying or soon-to-be-dying patients, clinging to life, their bodies decimated by nauseating chemotherapy, excoriating radiation, and disfiguring operative procedures.

So it was with a less-than-ideal attitude that I reported for my three-week stint on the leukemia and lymphoma service at The University of Iowa Hospital. Dr. Barnes, the attending oncologist, warmly greeted me and assigned a panel of patients to manage with the first-year internal medicine interns. Surprisingly, the patients were doing well, responding to treatment, and their case histories appeared to actually be *interesting*. An anti-nausea drug, ondansetron, had just been released, and astonishingly the chemotherapy-induced incidence of vomiting had declined to almost zero.

Over the subsequent three weeks, I sensed a gradual steady improvement in my medical skills. I learned about patients' medical histories, their life stories and families, and managed not only their malignancies but their entire medical care. While my knowledge base in internal medicine began to awaken and blossom, interacting with patients and families compassionately was an unexpected educational benefit. Unusual rashes, fevers, muscle pains, cardiac and kidney issues, shortness of breath and infections were daily issues which confronted our team. We worked hard to keep our patients healthy and in remission. I appreciated the opportunity to transform myself into a more complete physician during that brief moment in my medical education.

Midway through my rotation with the hematology-oncology team, I received a page about a new admission coming up from the emergency department. I read back the name from the unit clerk: Jackson Schmidt. Why did that name sound so familiar? After a few moments it came to me: *Is this my former professor from the College of Engineering?* Thirty minutes later, Dr. Schmidt arrived on the unit, confirming my suspicions. He had presented to the ED with significant fatigue, cough and low-grade fevers. Upon review of his chart and labs, he had a very elevated white blood cell count. Complicating matters was a multitude of abnormal, defective white cells seen under the microscope. The diagnosis was serious and concerning: chronic myelocytic leukemia (CML).

"Hi Dr. Schmidt, I don't know if you remember me, but I graduated in biomedical engineering a couple of years ago . . . we worked on a space symposium, remember?"

Dr. Schmidt gave me a tired smile in return. "Sure, nice to see you again, Bruce. Wish that we could've kept you in engineering, but it's good you stayed in Iowa City for more schooling."

I dutifully completed Dr. Schmidt's history and physical examination, and set up his initial care plan. It was pleasant to reconnect with him despite the troubling circumstances of our encounter. We reflected on the status of the College of Engineering, and talked about his wife of thirty-five years and their three children, all progressing well through college. He was in his late fifties and for the first time was seriously considering retirement. Although his diagnosis of leukemia was a serious one, in this modern age of medicine I remained optimistic about his chances for recovery and remission. I checked out with the first-year internal medicine resident, then went home for the evening, confident that we had the situation well in hand.

Our team for morning rounds reviewed Dr. Schmidt's case with our attending Dr. Barnes, then discussed our treatment plan with him and his wife. There was a thinly veiled apprehension in their eyes, which seemed to slightly dissipate in the face of our optimism for the care plan: an induction cycle of chemotherapy here in the hospital followed by several more cycles as an out-patient. The professor thoughtfully contemplated his treatment options in the methodical manner which befit his engineering background. After a nearly awkward pregnant pause, he quipped with a tired voice, "OK, let's do it."

Chemotherapy for cancer is the very definition of a scorched-earth battle, a Pyrrhic victory. Much like the historical wartime approach is to destroy the village in order to save it, chemotherapy employs toxic medications to obliterate the dangerous malignant cells. Unfortunately, many beneficial cells, including germ-fighting white blood cells, are also consumed in the process. Patients can develop not only the well-known hair loss, but also mouth sores, unusual infections, severe fatigue, strange rashes, nerve numbness and tingling, among countless other problems. Clinicians justify this strategy in that the patient has their "back against the wall," and action with cellular collateral damage is better than inaction against the marauding malignancies. I had already seen multiple leukemia patients muscle through these battles with inspired and dogged determination, and while weakened and emotionally spent, they also survived to fight on for another day.

Jackson initiated chemotherapy as a five-day induction, or introductory treatment, consisting of multiple medications. Like all of the other patients, the new anti-nausea medication kept him free from significant vomiting. Predictably his complete blood count labs over the coming days showed concerning precipitous declines in the red and white blood cell numbers. Red blood cells carry oxygen, which is vital to internal organ function. White blood cells form a first-line guardian defense against all types of infection, which in a debilitated patient can be life-threatening. Patients with severely depressed white blood cell counts are usually placed into isolation to protect them from these unusual microbial assaults. By day number five, Dr. Schmidt's red blood cell count was slightly down, but his white blood cell numbers were just a fraction of their baseline values; he was immediately and appropriately isolated.

At the end of a tumultuous week I called on him for morning rounds and was shocked at his appearance. He was drawn, haggard, pale and profoundly fatigued. In my six years of knowing him as a respected professor, I had never seen him in such a debilitated state.

"Hi Dr. Schmidt, how are you holdin' up after this challenging week?" I asked.

"Could be better, Bruce . . . I knew that this process would be difficult, but this was a lot harder than I expected."

"What problems are you noticing?"

"I'm totally wiped out, sweaty, my mouth hurts, I ache all over, through my muscles and deep into my bones. I've never felt this horrible in my entire life."

I performed a detailed physical examination on him. He was very diaphoretic, temperature elevated at 102.5 degrees, had a few red spots on his palate, and a mild, fine diffuse red rash. His lungs were clear on examination, but he also had a slight cough that was nagging him.

"Dr. Schmidt, I'm also concerned about you. Let me review your labs and exam findings with the team, and we will get things figured out, OK?"

"OK . . . sounds good."

I turned to leave, and as I almost reached the door, he had one additional question, the often profound patient "hand on the doorknob" inquiry as the doctor is leaving the room.

"Hey Doc . . . am I going to be OK?"

"Absolutely," I answered, trying to sound as confident and convincing as possible. I felt an abrupt, inexplicable ominous pang of doom about his long-term prognosis, and it bothered me in his atypical formality calling me Doc and not Bruce.

Within the hour, morning rounds wrapped up and everyone involved shared my deep concerns about Jackson. This was more than just a normal post-chemotherapy turn of events. When patients have low white counts and fever in cancer care, medically termed neutropenic fever, the workup is aggressive and detailed. Dr. Schmidt was started on three different antibiotics, and had blood, urine and sputum cultures obtained for analysis. These were all negative for bacteria. His chest X-ray was also normal. Still, he continued to press on with fever despite the antimicrobial nectar coursing through his veins and appropriate surveillance.

The following morning revealed a steady downward spiral in my former mentor's status. His fevers had not resolved, the white count was not improving, even after receiving a stimulating hormone, and now his blood pressures were declining. Dr. Schmidt was beginning to go into septic shock. Our team emergently transferred him to the medical ICU, and medications called pressors were started to help maintain his blood pressure. None of it was providing benefit, and it was beginning to dawn on the team and the family that this situation might be irreversible and untenable, seemingly unthinkable just one week ago.

After forty-eight hours of fluids, antibiotics and pressors, Jackson remained comatose, now intubated, on a ventilator, his heart, kidneys and liver in complete shutdown. Our care team reluctantly recognized the need to convene the family and discuss withdrawal of care. As a relatively green third-year medical student, I had not previously witnessed these types of discussions with families. Dr. Barnes was honest, compassionate and approachable in his discussions with Dr. Schmidt's family, but the conclusions of the family meeting were painful and clear: There was no hope left, it was time to let Jackson's spirit escape into the cosmos. Mrs. Schmidt and her children, while understandably shell-shocked, tearfully acquiesced to the withdrawal of these measures, and later that afternoon, Dr. Schmidt passed away.

The final pathology reports revealed the culprit: overwhelming sepsis, from a difficult-to-treat yeast infection in the bloodstream caused by *Candida tropicalis,* accompanied by an unforeseen transformation of his chronic leukemia to a lethal acute leukemia during the initiation of chemotherapy. Once these devastating building blocks of death were cemented into place, he never stood a chance.

I couldn't believe the tragic finality of it all. His treatment should have been a routine chemotherapy induction, followed by discharge to home, and close regular follow-ups and subsequent treatments. He was supposed to beat this cancer. He was relatively young, active, healthy and medically played by the rules. He ate well, exercised, kept regular checkups for physical examinations. It just wasn't fair. There was retirement, travels with his wife, grandchildren, hobbies; all of those dreams had permanently evaporated, never to be retrieved or recaptured.

Dr. Schmidt was an incredibly impactful patient to me: He was a mentor in my undergraduate engineering education, and I came to bond with him during his all-too-brief hospital stay. He confided in me his fears about what leukemia could do to his body and spirit. I felt a great sense of loss at his passing, and a twinge of gratitude for the last powerful lesson that he taught me that week about compassion and courage. In his darkest hour, he graciously called me "Doc," my professional title, a subtle acknowledging of my academic accomplishment.

None of those titles mattered now. Crushed and disillusioned, I walked off of the leukemia/lymphoma ward, down the wide hallway to the large windowed atrium at the end of the corridor. It was 5:00 p.m. on an October afternoon, and I felt an unexplained chill even as a brilliant orange sun was beginning its unrelenting descent toward the horizon. I despondently sank into an oversized brown leather chair, hoping to be mercifully swallowed up by its cushions and shielded from reality's unremitting harshness. I leaned forward and placed my heavy head into my waiting upturned hands for some feeble measure of support.

Suddenly, I was crying uncontrollably, salvos of sobbing punctuated by occasional quiet whimpering, thinking about the first special patient in my medical career to die. I felt disappointment and regret that despite all of our efforts, perhaps our team let him down that week. Already as a third-year medical student, I knew that this was the first of a countless multitude of unique people that would come into my medical world, become seriously ill, and ultimately pass away. Throughout my medical education, I was exhorted by my professors to learn as much as possible to positively serve my patients because my performance and decision-making were crucial. What has been an unexpected surprise through the years has been the transformational impacts *my patients* have impressed upon *my* spirit. I have grown to accept the unfortunate inevitabilities of physical frailty, clinical deterioration, culminating in death in medical practice. I remain thankful for the opportunities to enjoy the moments of good health and emotional contentment with my patients. My role is to offer my patients and their families not only intellectual insight, but also all of the compassion and insights that they richly deserve.

Almost too soon, the final week of my heme-onc rotation had approached. I felt smarter and more confident, but struggling emotionally to come to grips with losing Dr. Schmidt early on in the rotation. Dr. Barnes spotted my internal turmoil and took me aside one afternoon, his face conveying a genuine sense of concern for me.

"Bruce, I know that you really bonded with Dr. Schmidt. He was a unique individual. You'll never forget this educational moment in your medical career. But you also need to take those powerful clinical lessons and move on. There are other people that will need you, become seriously ill, and many more who will die. You not only need to do your best for them every single day, but also be *present in the moment with them.*"

With a poor attempt at a muffled sniffle, I thanked Dr. Barnes for his wisdom and insights. Even if I am sometimes bereft of clinical solutions for patients, I can always be supportive, compassionate and walk with them on their clinical journey.

Halloween fell during the last week of my time on the leukemia unit. I needed something to distract me and help me recover after losing my buddy. As a child, I always enjoyed dressing up in costume for Halloween. My mother lamented that she could never find or design a costume that would meet my exacting standards. I wasn't sure how the patients, staff and especially my attending physician would react to me showing up on the ward in festive regalia. After careful consideration, I decided on doing something simple—a headband with bunny ears, a painted pink nose and black eyeliner-placed whiskers. It was simple, yet whimsical, and if anyone had concerns about my appearance, I would simply remove the headband and wash my face.

October 31st arrived, and I applied my makeup and made my way to the University Hospital for my final day in oncology. I nervously made my appearance with my bunny garb, but from the look on everyone's faces I had nothing to worry about—I was a hit. One of the nurses made a cottontail for me out of a cluster of cotton balls. A patient, inspired by my efforts, emerged from his room with a puppy nose strapped on and makeshift dog ears. Dr. Barnes and my colleagues, seeing that it was tasteful and in good fun, all embraced the concept and were completely supportive. Over the course of the day, the bunny rabbit costume proved to be a good icebreaker and served to dismantle some of the virtual walls that exist between patients and care teams. It was a memorable professional experience; to this day, I wear my bunny ears, pink nose and whiskers to work at Easter, and dress up in a costume for Halloween. It has inspired me to be a transformational person both for myself and the patients under my care.

Mid-July in Iowa can be warm and beautiful, but also oppressively humid and sticky. I spent the summer after my sophomore year of college getting into solid physical condition riding my bike nearly every day around my hometown of Oskaloosa. After completing my ubiquitous summer job, I would spend an hour or two vigorously propelling my bicycle over the smoothly paved quiet county highways through the rolling hills of the countryside, often passing multiple old strip-mining sites. At the beginning of the twentieth century, these deep pits churned out vast quantities of bituminous coal, which helped power locomotives and the machinery that advanced the progress of a nation. For the last fifty years all of the mines have remained quiet and shuttered, with no signs of any resurgence of the coal-harvesting culture.

I contemplated how coal began as simple prehistoric vegetation, only to undergo a metamorphic transformation from millions of years of pressure and darkness into a blackened carbon treasure. Through the generations, many of my ancestors, friends and descendants have taken life's challenges and produced their own elegant personal revolution. Whether recovering from a loss or learning something new, I reminded myself to power through the depressing uncertainty in hopes of arriving at a transmutative, glorious destination.

CHAPTER 8

REDNESS

Whether posted on a ubiquitous octagonal stop sign or the glaring flashing lights posted at a railroad crossing, the color red never fails to garner attention. In the medical world, reddish discoloration often symbolizes a significant change in a patient's condition. Doctors encounter shades of crimson with hemorrhaging patients, skin infections, inflamed joints, and even an adorable child with a high fever. It is a diagnostic finding which is difficult to overlook, and when identified, requires prompt evaluation and appropriate treatment.

Carly Jensen was a cute three-year-old girl, forever enshrined into my professional memory, as she was the first baby I delivered as an attending physician. Her parents were devoted and supportive, but one day they came to me with a sense of frustration. For several weeks she struggled with a severe, persistent groin rash, and saw a fellow pediatrician in the office. He appropriately started her on an anti-fungal cream for presumptive candidal yeast dermatitis, the number-one cause of diaper rash in young children. However, despite completing two weeks of the cream treatment, the rash had not improved.

"Hi guys, it's Dr. Bruce," I began cheerfully. "Sounds like you have a bad diaper rash that needs a recheck today."

"I'll say," Carly's Mom responded sadly, "this is the worst rash I've ever seen on her. We've tried all kinds of over-the-counter creams, and the prescription medication we got from Dr. DeGroot last week. Nothing helps at all, I can't believe it."

"Any other new lotions, detergents, perfumes, new foods in the diet?" I asked curiously.

"No—everything with that has been the same," replied her father.

Carly's examination was normal, with the exception of her buttocks and groin area. There, conspicuously displayed in an angry butterfly pattern, was an intense vermillion rash with evidence of childlike scratching. It was one of the worst-looking diaper rashes that I had ever witnessed in clinical practice. She had small dots around the rash, the so-called satellite lesions which are diagnostic of a yeast infection. *But why was this rash not improving?* Severe nonhealing diaper rashes usually can be traced to a couple of unique causes: One was zinc deficiency, which was quite rare in children in the developed world, and juvenile diabetes, which was all-too common in primary care. At that moment, I remembered that Carly's father was a Type I diabetic since the age of fourteen. It became clear what the next step should be in Carly's evaluation.

"Guys, we need to check a blood glucose on Carly. I'm concerned because of the severity of the rash and the difficulty we're having getting it to clear."

OK Doc, sounds like as good a plan as any, especially since for two weeks we have gotten nowhere," Mrs. Jensen replied with rising apprehension of a possible serious medical diagnosis. "I sure hope that it's not diabetes . . . one insulin-dependent diabetic in our family is enough."

I made a delicate attempt to reassure the family, although I was worried about what we might find on Carly's evaluation. "I agree, but given the circumstances and family history, I feel this is the next logical step."

Carly went to the lab to get her finger poked to check a blood glucose. Unfortunately, on two consecutive tries, the meter simply read, "HIGH." This was a bad sign, as it indicates the level is too high to be measured by meter, with a glucose in excess of 600mg/dL, and normal levels tend to be around 100mg/dL. As a result, we sent Carly to the ER at Children's Hospital, where her serum blood glucose was 900mg/dL, unfortunately a new diagnosis of Type I juvenile diabetes.

With her father's support she started on injectable insulin. While the diaper rash rapidly resolved, her medical issues were just beginning: Type I diabetes is a lifelong struggle with glucose control and preventing secondary complications. At a recent adolescent wellness visit, Carly appeared to be weathering the storm surprisingly well. Her father strove to be a good role model with his diabetic control—I hoped that Carly would learn from his experiences and remain compliant with her treatments.

Other cases of redness are extremely peculiar and are not so easily diagnosable. As a senior resident I began my shift at

Children's Hospital emergency department on a warm, muggy July evening. The unit was already humming, with fevers, asthma exacerbations, and a myriad of broken bones from the daily exploits of the daring youth of metropolitan Milwaukee.

I checked over the board listing the patients, which was already jam-packed, and grabbed the next chart in the queue. I pored over the top line, which listed the Chief Complaint, sometimes "CC" for short. When the pace of the patient inflow became unwieldy, the nurse's written reasons for the visit became quite truncated. My first patient's paperwork simply stated "Red, hot left cheek."

Intrigued with a novel presenting symptom, I entered the bright, clean room in the corner of a long hallway. I greeted the parents and was introduced to Maria, a pleasant, quiet two-year-old Hispanic toddler.

"Hi there, I'm Dr. Bruce," I said cheerfully. "Oh dear, it looks like you have a very red cheek." The child and her parents seemed pleasant, not alarmed nor distressed by the current circumstances. Her mother spoke first.

"Yes Doctor, she was fine yesterday, then woke up this morning with a very bright red cheek. It feels a little warm today."

"Has she had any fevers, chills, sore throat, appetite changes, ear pain or any other unusual body rashes.?"

Her father chimed in. "No, she hasn't had any of those problems."

"Any runny or stuffy nose, cough, shortness of breath?"

"No, not at all," her mother replied.

On initial examination, the pretty young toddler looked alert and playful, and her vital signs were stable, without a sign of fever.

In fact, the only salient feature on her physical exam was a prominent warm, red left cheek area. Her eardrums and posterior pharynx were normal. There was no generalized body rash to suggest a viral syndrome. I ran through a list of potential diagnoses in my mind: *Fifth disease, trauma, abuse, cellulitis, urticaria, contact dermatitis,* but I was unclear of a definitive cause of her problem. All signs seemed to point toward a classic diagnosis of buccal cellulitis—a bacterial infection in the skin of the left cheek.

Dr. Hameed Hassan was the senior attending physician working that night in the emergency department. Dr. Hassan was a veteran, established board-certified pediatric emergency medicine physician, whose parents emigrated from Egypt decades prior. He had a reputation for being a tough but fair colleague and teacher, and was a fierce advocate for his residents if their capabilities were challenged in any way by any outside specialty physician. He had a tightly clipped salt-and-pepper mustache, and touches of gray had begun to appear in his jet-black hair near his temples, which framed his olive complexion.

I politely grabbed Dr. Hassan's attention, and in ordered detail presented my case and its related findings. As I spoke, I felt my confidence growing in that I had appropriately evaluated and diagnosed my patient.

"I believe that this child has buccal cellulitis, and we should begin her on a ten-day course of dicloxacillin, with plans to see her primary pediatrician in two weeks."

But Dr. Hassan appeared to be neither moved nor impressed by my presentation assessment or my recommendations, and he remained quiet and thoughtful after I had completed my patient summary.

"Hmmm—usually the cause of unilateral [one-sided] buccal cellulitis is the bacterium *Haemophilus influenzae*. We have been immunizing against that for the last ten years, so it doesn't seem like that would be the cause. Are her immunizations up to date?" In the pediatric setting, it was always critical to verify immunization status. I had already discussed this with Maria's parents—her vaccinations were all current and in order. He didn't make any further queries, and nonverbally indicated that he had heard enough and was ready to see our young lady for himself.

My confidence was now slightly shaken, but I continued to cling to my belief that once Dr. Hassan assessed Maria, he would see the diagnosis my way and I would be vindicated.

Dr. Hassan followed me into the patient examination room, introduced himself, and commenced with an abbreviated assessment of his own, building on some of the identical information that I had asked previously. His examination revealed the same features that I had identified, with no additional or unusual findings that I had understated or missed. Surely, now he was convinced that my diagnosis and treatment plan was the avenue of choice for Maria.

Instead, he finished checking Maria over, primly straightened up, and asked the parents an odd, but ultimately profound question:

"Have you been giving your child popsicles?"

What? Where was this line of questioning going? I thought to myself, *this seems ridiculous and makes absolutely no sense.* My mind was permeated by a sense of incredulity and was intrigued by how the parents would react to this left-field question.

Surely this path of inquiry would be exposed for its lunacy and peculiarity.

But instead of seeing parental confusion and consternation, I was shocked by their agreement and affirmation.

"Why yes, the weather has been so very hot, so we have been giving her a couple of popsicles per day . . . she really likes their sweet taste," responded the mother. "Was that the wrong thing to do for her?" She was genuinely concerned, with a twinge of guilt that she may have unintentionally done something that could generate a health problem.

Dr. Hassan kindly reassured the parents. "Why no, it's simply that she is not old enough to have a popsicle right now. She isn't able to move the popsicle around in her mouth like she should, so the popsicle stays in one spot inside her cheek, and she gets a localized area of frostbite and temporary damage to the tissues. I would wait on the popsicles for another a year or so, and just use some ibuprofen as needed for pain. She will make a full recovery—don't feel bad, this happens more frequently to children than you realize."

He then turned to me and smiled. His sable-brown eyes were constructive and warm. "Bruce—this is a classic case of popsicle panniculitis, thermal damage to the fatty tissues of the cheek from the cold popsicle being held stationary in the mouth for an extended period of time. Since the popsicle remains confined to the same place, the cold is concentrated all in one location. Can you please have the nurse give the family their checkout information?"

Now I felt a redness in *my* cheek, but mine was on both sides, and arose because I was embarrassed not only by my misdiagnosis, but also that I was not even close to figuring out Maria's actual medical problem. It was not a great way to begin my emergency room shift.

Quietly and somewhat abashedly, I finished up with Maria and her parents, then plunged into the remainder of my eight-hour shift. The evening otherwise progressed well, and I had a plethora of cases that I diagnosed and treated appropriately. Midnight arrived, and after completing all of my charts, I quietly walked off to the locker room to change out of my scrubs and head home for a good night's sleep. Maria's case still loomed large in my mind. Although it was not a life-threatening issue, I internally felt angry at my diagnostic inadequacy and inability to project my medical self-assuredness toward my patients.

After I closed my locker door a bit too hard, preparing to leave, I turned and came in to contact with a pair of eyes. They were the same pair of warm brown irises that had taught me earlier in the shift.

Dr. Hassan spoke first. "Bruce, I could tell you were disappointed in not getting the diagnosis on that kid with panniculitis. Don't be so hard on yourself. Remember, I have twenty years of clinical experience in medicine that you don't have yet. Also, there was a picture and description of this very case in the last edition of *Nelson's Textbook of Pediatrics.* Just remember—medicine is a never-ending learning process. Keep working hard, you'll get there. You have all of the ingredients to become a great doctor."

I was humbled and mumbled an unacceptably audible "Thanks." In a flash, he smiled pleasantly, shook my hand and disappeared. Having now accumulated twenty years of my own medical foundation and memories, I never forgot the significance of that patient encounter and its deeper ramifications. In cases where my diagnosis was incorrect, it remains important to identify it, learn from it, and then move forward.

Redness doesn't discriminate based on age; it affects the old and young to an equivalent degree. On Tuesday mornings, I complete my rounds at the Alexian Village Retirement Community, seeing independent, assisted living, and nursing home patients. I enjoy the interactions with my geriatric brethren, learning about their life histories and their families in the context of providing them with quality health care and emotional support.

Dorothy Sanders was a lovely eighty-eight-year-old lady who I saw in the nursing home area for a routine follow-up visit. However, she noted an acute problem—a three-day history of an increasing pain in her lower back area, extending on one side into the right buttock area. She denied any history of trauma or falls recently, but she had become increasingly irritable and tearful, so I knew that this level of pain was bothering this normally stoic woman. A few years prior, we diagnosed her with a subtle lower back and pelvic fracture, which presented in a similar fashion.

I examined Dorothy, and she had some moderate lower back and right buttock pain on exam. She had no numbness or any other alarming neurological findings which could suggest a spinal cord crisis. However, during my exam I neglected to raise up her shirt and lower her pants to check her skin directly, an oversight which would prove to be significant. I made a provisional diagnosis of myofascial strain versus osteoarthritis and moved along with my scheduled patient evaluations.

Forty-eight hours elapsed, and I had returned to the retirement community to complete teaching rounds with the family medicine residents. Dorothy's nurse, Cheryl, caught my attention and politely approached me to request some assistance.

"Dr. Rowe, can you check on Dorothy again today? She's really having a great deal of pain. You and I both know that she normally doesn't complain about anything, so this seems weird."

"Sure, I will get over there and reexamine her later this morning," I replied agreeably, not giving it a second thought. Maybe she just needed an increase in her Tylenol pain medication, or a referral over to physical therapy for further treatment and pain management. I finished up with my students and made my way over to the wing where Dorothy resided. She was just finishing her lunch, so I wheeled her over to her room to perform a reassessment.

"Dorothy, is your pain really bad now?"

"Yes Doc, it's worse than when I had that broken back a few years ago."

"How bad is it, and what does it feel like?"

"Oh, it's pretty bad, and it feels like tingling and burning . . ."

Tingling and burning? That doesn't sound like muscle strain or arthritis, this sounds more like neuropathic pain. This type of discomfort is related to inflamed nerve endings deep within the skin. Other than some buttock burning and tingling, her motor strength in her legs and neurological exam remained normal. Finally, I completed the step in the physical exam that I neglected to execute two days ago: I moved her clothing out of the way to examine the skin directly. Here was where I belatedly identified the culprit: multiple angry clusters of vermillion vesicular blisters cascading from the lower back and across the right mid-posterior buttock, following a nerve root distribution in a very distinct fashion. *Crap! It's shingles! Man, I forgot to take a minute to simply take a look at the skin surface. If I had, surely I'd have seen this two days ago.* Shingles, or herpes zoster, occurs when the normally dormant chicken pox virus reactivates and attacks a vulnerable isolated nerve root. Feeling sheepish and contrite, I notified Dorothy of my findings, and promptly started her on an antiviral treatment and prednisone. She made a full recovery, and fortunately did not experience any of the chronic post-inflammatory pain that plagues many of these patients.

Once again, a red cheek educated me about an important tenet in primary care medicine: *A physical examination always starts with inspection.* In the process of not directly visualizing the skin in the region of concern, I became misled about Dorothy's diagnosis and ended up with an incorrect medical assessment. Subsequently, for every relevant physical examination that I perform, I now complete an evaluation of the skin surface. My embarrassment was tempered by the ultimate realization that my initial professional folly improved my medical practice.

The term "red herring," or misleading and spurious information, is frequently bandied about in our lexicon, but especially in political and literary spheres of society. However, as a physician I have witnessed many clinical presentations which often do not make sense on first assessment. Occasionally they may take me in a completely incorrect diagnostic direction before I right the ship into an accurate orientation. The ruby fish can be insidious, and the implications of being misdirected range from a minor delay in diagnosis to life-threatening complications and death. Past tricky patient experiences, both rewarding and unpleasant, often prove to be the most instructional moments in medicine.

Pamela was a very sweet, independent-living seventy-five-year-old elderly white female whom I had treated for the last several years. She was a retired medical laboratory technician, so she always gave an excellent accounting of her symptoms. Over the last few years, we had treated her for an irregular heartbeat called atrial fibrillation, elevated cholesterol levels, and moderate depression. After an uneventful period of several months, my concerns were raised when she presented with a recent onset of unusual symptoms.

"Hi Pam, nice to see you today. How've you been feeling since our last visit?" I asked cheerfully.

"I don't know, Doc, I just have a lot of aches and pains all over, it lasts all day, and now it's hard for me to go on my walks and get stuff done like I used to." There was a sense of tiredness and concern emanating in her voice that was atypical compared to other encounters.

"Have you had a cold or flu over the last few weeks or months?"

"No."

"Any recent travel or contact with someone who has been seriously ill?"

"Nope."

"Has your mood been OK, not slipping back into any depression issues?"

"Mood's been good . . . no real problems there, the medication you gave me for that has really helped."

"I know you do the Senior Fit aerobics. You're not overdoing it there, are you?"

"Not right now . . . in fact, I haven't been there for weeks, and it hasn't made any difference in the soreness at all. Tylenol and ibuprofen haven't helped at all either. This is really a weird thing for me." Her countenance exposed an internal spinning of the wheels in her head, trying to discern what could possibly be amiss.

Her examination was similarly murky and unrevealing, only showing several nonspecific areas of some sore muscles throughout her body. However, when I reviewed her medical list, I hit paydirt—she was taking atorvastatin, a cholesterol-lowering medication of which a major side effect was myalgias—an achiness of her muscles.

"Pam, I think I got it pegged here . . . you've been on this new cholesterol medication for the last several months, and that coincides almost exactly with the timing of when your muscle soreness began. If we stop this medication immediately and complete a short course of physical therapy, I think that you'll be back to your old self."

She brightened. "Oh thanks, Doc . . . you're the best, I knew that I could count on you!"

"Sure Pam, see you in three to four weeks, OK?"

Feeling confident of my diagnostic conclusions, I expectantly looked forward to a follow-up visit with corresponding clinical improvement. In retrospect, I should have remained on guard for my intellectual hubris: Sometimes my premature self-congratulatory thoughts are interrupted by the alternative true medical cause lurking in the background.

One month elapsed, and Pam followed up in my office. I could tell immediately by the reflective gaze in her eyes and slouched body language that things were not progressing well for her.

I initiated the break in the uncomfortable silence. "I guess I don't even need to ask how the month went, I can tell from the look on your face that it hasn't been worth shouting about."

Pam gathered herself to reply. She wasn't angry at me or the situation, rather she appeared resigned and disappointed. "Nope, still hurt all over. I really thought we had this figured out last month, was there something we overlooked?"

"I did as well . . . I was sure that it was your cholesterol medication, but if that were the case, your pains should be getting better by now."

In rethinking a diagnosis, a good approach to take is like you lost something, and attempting to relocate it. Simply retrace your steps, retake a medical history, repeat your physical exam and hopefully you will find the cause of the problem missed on the first attempt.

Think, Bruce! She said it was a soreness, and it is steadily worsening with time, and worse with activity . . . that means it could be a rheumatologic, or autoimmune process! Now this was something worth exploring. I checked for eye redness, joint swelling of her hands, unusual rashes—nope, nothing remarkable there. Next, I checked her muscle achiness and soreness again. It now was primarily located over her shoulder and hip areas, and when I asked her to describe in further detail, she revealed it was a stiffness. At this point, I began to believe that we were now on the cusp of something medically significant. One last area to check: I palpated both her left and right temple areas, feeling for tenderness over her temporal arteries. She had mild tenderness there, too, then she volunteered that her jaw hurt when struggling with chewy foods. A set of lab tests provided the final piece in the puzzle—her erythrocyte sedimentation rate (ESR), a key measure of total body inflammation, was sky-high, at 76 mm/hr (Normal < 20).

Hallelujah! Now I felt like we had the answer. It had nothing to do with the lipid-lowering medication at all. Rather, it was an autoimmune condition known as Polymyalgia Rheumatica (PMR)/Temporal Arteritis, a tricky diagnosis in elderly patients. The treatment of choice is prednisone, often in higher doses. When I outlined the diagnosis and treatment recommendations to Pam, her face broke into a smile and she simply stated, "Go for it!" We started her on prednisone 20 mg daily, tapering down by a 1 mg per day every month, for a total of twenty months. This time, we planned to get back together in a few weeks for a recheck.

Two weeks later, a beaming Pamela showed up in my office, and it was clear that we had rounded the corner. "Thanks so much, Doc! Your persistence and good listening skills paid off . . . I feel like a million bucks now!" Watching her leave the office, I swear that she made a slight skip in her steps.

In early August between high school graduation and college, my friends went out on a nearby lake for a boating and water-skiing trip. The weather was beautiful, with bright, brilliant sunshine bathing us all day as we joyfully launched our skis over the rolling waves, being towed behind the powerful speedboat.

All too quickly the daylight began its predestined surrender to the encroaching night. As we anchored and consumed a late picnic dinner in the boat, I glanced toward the western horizon to witness a spectacular sunset, with its warm and perfect reflection on the placid lake waters. A polychromatic palette of reds, pinks and purples greeted my gaze, distracting me from the slight evening chill, a subtle harbinger of the autumn months to come. High rose-colored cirrus clouds stretched toward the horizon like warm cotton candy. At the time I contemplated that I was leaving my buddies to attend my freshman year of college in a couple of short weeks, sadly realizing our inevitably diverging life pathways. Over the years, as I regularly encounter redness in life, whether in the office, emotionally or in a beautiful landscape, it serves as a sign that something is brewing in the air, for better or for worse.

CHAPTER 9

CRITICAL

Constructive criticism, delivered by senior experienced staff physicians, with the expectation that junior residents and medical students accept and improve behaviors, is the hallmark of medical education. After all, people's lives are depending on a physician's knowledge and professionalism. Didactic teaching, public scrutiny and adversarial feedback are essential components in perfecting clinical skills. When presented in an encouraging fashion, these experiences can serve as a valuable growth opportunity. Senior staff doctors who deploy comments in a belittling or condescending manner can undermine a medical trainee's confidence, questioning their skills and career choice.

Medical students, upon entering their third year of graduate training, embark on a variety of monthly clinical work environments referred to as rotations. Rotations expose third-year trainees to a comprehensive variety of health-care experiences. All students undergo a complete yearlong clinical learning atmosphere, helping to facilitate an ultimate choice of medical specialty. Every medical student on rounds has their medical knowledge plumbed by senior residents and attending physicians, a process colloquially referred to as *pimping* due to its intimidating nature. Some examples of questions that my senior physician colleagues grilled me about included the following:

What is the LDH pleural fluid to serum ratio which differentiates transudates versus exudates?

What are the Ranson criteria in acute pancreatitis?

Can you name the four causes of ST segment elevation on an electrocardiogram?

Typically the aspiring doctor caught in the pimping trap has three responses at their disposal: First, completely knowing the answer and responding with crisp appropriateness. Second, having a general idea of the gist of the question and attempting to construct some semblance of an effective response. Finally, drawing a complete mental blank, struggling mightily to not appear completely clueless or ignorant. Every trainee has faced all three of these clinical scenarios throughout medical school. Reveling in your knowledge and accepting your shortcomings is key to survival. Occasionally, a sympathetic resident standing behind the attending will mouth the answer to you, a sort of academic lifeline. Fortunately, I could confide to classmates my misery and embarrassment when questioning got tough.

At the end of my third year I was placed in a neurology rotation on the stroke unit at the University of Iowa Hospital. Each morning the students were expected to report to the attending doctor on the status of admissions to the unit overnight. It had been my first call night on the service, and Dr. Carson, the staff neurologist, came to the floor at 8:00 a.m. for rounds. He was reasonably pleasant but didn't suffer fools gently.

"Alright, any new admissions from the overnight to present to me this morning?" he briefly queried.

Recalling my recent, busy general internal medicine rotation, I presented quickly as possible, like we were taught previously. "Mrs. Schwartz is a sixty-two-year-old white female who presented with aphasia, right-sided facial droop, and right-sided weakness which was confirmed on physical examination. She has high cholesterol and was a former smoker. No other non-neurological findings on physical examination. Her CT scan showed—"

"Wait—what are you doing?" he interjected.

"Presenting the case to you. I thought that you wan—"

"No no no! Please present the History and Physical in a complete and organized fashion, start at the beginning and go through the entire case like you were taught and are supposed to do on this service. Thank you . . ."

Embarrassed, I felt the sympathetic stares of my fellow medical students and residents bearing down upon me. I mentally retraced my steps, looked at my handwritten H&P note, and like reading a boring shopping list dutifully summarized my case presentation. It was an unnecessary prolongation, a waste of time full of extraneous unnecessary details; but it was what attending requested, and that reality took precedent over all others. Upon completion of my droning clinical novella, Dr. Carson primly straightened himself, tightened his necktie, half-smiled and said, "See there, Bruce? That's how I want the cases on this rotation presented. Do you people understand that? I want the complete story every time, on every patient! *Comprende?*"

"Yes, sir," the entire care team murmured in muffled response, awkwardly shifting their feet in unison. No one likes being the sacrificial lamb on a medical teaching service. However, I needed to develop constructive responses to appropriate feedback, even if it was delivered in a somewhat gruff manner.

As springtime approached, the end of the third-year clerkship grind loomed on the horizon. Hopeful and excited, I was flying high and brimming with confidence. I had completed a rotation on our psychiatry service, receiving an honors grade. My girlfriend Laura came in for Valentine's Day weekend from Philadelphia, and we got engaged. Everything in my life seemed to be falling into place. At last I would move past the required rotations and begin my fourth year of medical school. In the homestretch as a senior medical student, classification M4, I would able to embark on some training experiences of specific interest to me in my future career. All that remained was the six-week mountainous challenge of general surgery.

I was under no false illusions that the month-and-a-half experience of a surgical endeavor would not be significantly difficult. My classmates described getting up at 4:15 a.m., rounding on patients at 5:00 a.m., morning rounds with the team at 6:00 a.m., beginning a full days' worth of operations by 7:00 a.m., postoperative examinations, working up new admissions, and culminating with evening rounds. If there were no emergent surgical cases, the day would end at around 8:00 or 9:00 p.m., only to recur during the earliest hours of the following early-morning twilight. Adding insult to injury of this grueling physical process was the frequent emotional stresses of constructive criticism devolving into negative feedback, belittling and often pointless in nature. Surgical teams tended to be very hierarchal during that era, and the anger and hostility tended to run downhill, from attending, to senior resident, junior resident, senior med student, and ultimately down to the lowest life-form of the team, the third-year medical student.

The first morning of my surgical rotation arrived deceptively quiet and early, on a cold, snowy Monday right after my blissful Valentine's Day engagement weekend. Laura had already flown back to Philly, so I was alone once again. Five of my fellow third-year students and I were assigned to Team 2, which was known for somewhat friendlier attending physicians—my first break. However, the wildcard on your surgical team was who served as your chief resident. The chief was a fifth-year surgical resident, on the brink of moving on to fellowship or full-fledged clinical practice.

A chief resident could make or break a young student's rotational experience; a good one often was friendly, supportive and committed to developing and educating young aspiring physicians. It was even better yet if they had a young family to get home to in the evening, which often meant efficient late-afternoon rounds and an early dismissal home. Bad and/or mean chief residents were the worst. They possessed a terrible combination of arrogance, lack of commitment to teaching, excessively delegating responsibility and unnecessarily degrading students for trivial reasons. Unpopular and mean chiefs forced students to stay at the hospital late into the evening for pointless rounding, or required them to perform other worthless tasks, so-called "scut work."

Although I somewhat enjoyed the work involved with general surgery, I never visualized myself in a future career as a general surgeon. The long hours and the significant physical and emotional demands of the specialty were undesirable. However, I also realized that in order to get a good grade and advance to fourth-year status, I would need to perform confidently on the surgical wards and in the OR.

After our first morning sign-out session of the rotation, we linked up with our upper-level residents. By this stage in the third year, our classmates had clued us in on which residents were excellent and those who were nightmarish. Our team had a first-year surgical intern, a third-year resident and, finally, a fifth-year chief resident. I didn't know the lower-level residents on this rotation, but when our fifth-year came over to meet us, my heart sank . . . Sheila Devlin, arguably the meanest chief on any service at the U. She was awkwardly tall, pale and tired-looking, with a drab simple short haircut, and she wore no makeup. She looked chronically unhappy, her tight thin lips essentially frozen into a frowning position. Sheila also was an intelligent and talented surgeon, it just didn't always translate into warmth or empathy. I put on my best poker face to hide my disappointment with my assignment, but Dr. Devlin didn't give us much time to contemplate our fates.

"Alright you fleas," she sputtered, poorly concealing her frustration and lack of confidence in our abilities. "Talk with the intern, get your patient assignments, go round on them, get to know them, and figure out the treatment plan for the day. We need to meet in about an hour to review patient status and get started on today's OR schedule. I need thorough assessments and complete evaluations, got it?" For no good reason, her icy stare fixated on me, unblinking, devoid of any level of positivity. "You—what the hell's your name?" she inquired with a thin veneer of hostility.

"Bruce Rowe, M3 student," I replied clearly and diplomatically.

"What speciality do you want to go into after graduation?" she countered.

"I don't know—maybe orthopedic surgery . . ."

"Hope that you're smart, good with your hands, and have a lot of confidence," she answered. "You're gonna need all three to make it in that competitive field, and I'm not sure that describes you."

Oh no! She's dishing out insults, trying to make me look bad already! So how do I respond to this attack?

"Yes, I hope so," I replied with a too-deferential tone, already my first mistake. In the dog-eat-dog, cutthroat world of the surgeons, I needed to immediately project strength and confidence. I quickly sensed my emotional oversight and realized that I had obtained a powerful malignant adversary on my team for the next month and a half. She seemed to despise all of us, but she reserved the most hostile invective for me every day.

A typical day on my surgical rotation would proceed like this: I would awaken every morning at an insane hour and make my way to the hospital by about 5:00 a.m. After rounding on my patients by myself, the team would gather for our initial morning report. Every day Dr. Devlin would formulate a new and unique way to embarrass me in front of the group. There was always a piece of information or insight that she wanted that I didn't have readily at my disposal. After my latest episode of humiliation I would valiantly attempt to improve my performance, only to be accused of a new offense at the next session of rounding.

"Bruce—what was the 24-hour I and O [Intake and Output] for Mrs. Hughes?"

"3500 cc in, 2500 cc out."

"How much from the drain?"

"125 cc in the last 24 hours."

"How much from the drain the last 8 hours?"

"I don't have that information."

"How can you not check this? I cannot believe you sometimes, and that you are a third-year . . . I need to know the latest 8-hour outputs on all of the patients, understand?"

"Yes Dr. Devlin," I replied too contritely. If I were a dog, my tail would be curled up between my hind legs, virtually fused to my lower body. It was a terrifying progressive feedback loop: The more I appeared sorry and apologetic, increasingly angrier and relentless she became. The vacuum of my fear became completely filled with her ego, brimming with derision and hostility. My fellow students and even lower-level surgical residents looked at me empathetically, feeling my internal agony but knowing that in the pyramidal world of surgical command, they could only remain silent.

In the operating room, she spared no opportunity to criticize my inability to answer a complicated anatomical question or deride my technical skills. Despite my solid manual dexterity under normal circumstances, my hands often felt uncontrolled, visibly shaking in the blinding-hot presence of her cruel scrutiny.

"Alright Bruce, place those subcuticular sutures to close up that wound . . . No! That's not how I want you to hold the needle driver . . . Evert the tissues, even bites on both sides . . . Good God! Do you really think that you're surgeon material? . . . I can't believe your awkwardness with your hands!"

With slightly watery eyes, I looked over at the attending physician, Dr. Timothy Criswell, for possible support and salvation. In the narrow zone between his head covering and surgical mask I thought I detected a slight eyeroll and his irises staring up toward the heavens as if to say, "What's her problem now?" But of course in accordance with the unspoken surgical training code, he said nothing. I remained quiet and suppressed any tears, trying to maintain focus on the patient, learning about surgery and refining my technical skills.

With one week remaining on my hellish surgical journey, I was at a loss about my predicament. I was being harshly criticized daily much more adversely and personally compared to my third-year compatriots. Though the calendar showed winter giving way to spring, I felt an autumnal despondency sliding into a chilly depression. *Maybe I am not cut out to be any type of surgeon, or even a doctor. Do I have any recourse to address this incredibly stressful and difficult work situation?*

Briefly I considered filing a complaint against her with the residency director, but ultimately I decided against it. There were too many potential adverse consequences to that action. I risked being labeled as a troublemaker, weak, and not cut out for the normal stresses of surgical practice. A vindictive chief resident who was called out on the carpet could easily make life even more miserable for me. Far better for me to tough things out for another week, get my average grade for the rotation, walk away, and hopefully never work on a general surgery service again.

Over time I have felt my attitude soften somewhat with respect to the challenging time I spent with my general surgical brethren. Dr. Devlin taught me the importance of being prepared, projecting confidence, and remaining strong in the presence of intense, withering criticism, warranted or not. To her credit, she was proven correct—*I wasn't cut out to be a surgeon.* I also realized that despite my dedication and kindness, there would always be people who simply would not like me, nor be in my corner. While a difficult concept to accept, it also presents a stark reality, and I no longer excessively ruminate on how to improve an unsalvageable interpersonal situation. As a fiery hot furnace hardens steel, the stress of harsh criticism, while uncomfortable, has made me a better person and more effective doctor.

One summer evening, I was called into the ER as the second-year family medicine resident on the inpatient medical service for an admission. Annie was sixty-two years old, but looked somewhat older, related to overtanning from countless days spent on a sun-soaked golf course. Her skin had a medium-brown texture, and was excessively leathery throughout all her sun-exposed areas. The presenting complaint written on the front of the chart said simply, "Extreme Weakness." Intrigued with the vague and nonspecific symptom presentation, I knocked and politely entered the patient room.

"Hi there, I'm Dr. Rowe, I hear that you've been feeling weak and tired recently."

"Yessir, that's an understatement. I was fine until the last week when the wheels began to come off," Annie replied quietly. Even simple conversing seemed to be an effort for her. "I feel so weak, I can't even lift my head up and can barely move my muscles."

This appeared to be more significant than run-of-the-mill weakness issues. She was legitimately incapacitated by the extent of her muscular dysfunction.

"Any headaches, visual changes, numbness, tingling, difficulty speaking or swallowing recently?" I queried.

"No—I haven't had any of those issues at all," she feebly responded.

"Any new medications, travel, chemical exposures, recent viral illness?"

She answered in the negative to all of those questions.

Her physical examination findings were unremarkable, with the exception of diminished deep tendon reflexes throughout and moderate weakness in all major muscle groups. No other abnormalities were present on the initial assessment, so it was time to begin the diagnostic side of the workup. She was understandably alarmed when I referred to her significant fatigue, decreased muscle tone and abnormal reflexes.

"Doctor, am I going to be OK?" she meekly asked.

"Yes ma'am, we're going to get this figured out for you today."

Potential diagnoses for Annie included Guillain-Barre Syndrome, atypical stroke, hemiplegic migraine, infection, B12 or folic acid deficiency, toxin, or some degenerative neurologic condition. The head CT scan was negative—my first piece of good news of the night. Her hemogram showed a normal white blood cell count, reducing our suspicion of infection. While contemplating the need to perform a lumbar puncture, a significant diagnostic finding dramatically emerged on her metabolic lab panel: severe hypokalemia, with a potassium level profoundly decreased to around 1.7 mEq/L (normal level is 3.5–5.0).

This appeared to be the cause of my patient's severe motor weakness, but the larger question was why? According to our sporadic records, she was not on any medications, and had no other major health issues. Was she intentionally or inadvertently withholding a critical piece of health information? After writing orders for the ICU and to treat her depleted potassium, I returned to Annie's room in the hope of solving the mystery of how she suddenly ended up in such a debilitated state.

"Annie, your potassium stores are critically low," conveying ominous tension. "Do you know how this could have happened? Any unusual diets? Any recent vomiting or diarrhea episodes?"

She displayed a flash of narrowing defensiveness in her eyes, which then subsided to a widening sense of embarrassment. "Well, a few weeks ago, I received a shipment of water pills through the mail from Mexico. My legs swell up so badly, and I just had to do something about it." She presented me with the names of two potent diuretics she was taking without a prescription or doctor's supervision via a simple mail order procedure. The meds were furosemide 40 mg twice per day and hydrochlorothiazide 50 mg twice per day. These were hefty diuretic doses, even for a person with a true water-retention problem.

I was incredulous, attempting to hide my frustration and sense of indignation. "Annie, these are very powerful water pills, you need to take them under a doctor's care with close electrolyte monitoring. You now have a life-threatening potassium depletion problem as a result."

"I know it was the wrong thing to do, Doc, but I just needed to do something about all of my excess fluid, it was driving me crazy."

This was a discussion best held when the patient was in better condition to engage in constructive dialogue. "Alright, let's get you upstairs, we'll correct these issues and talk again tomorrow."

The treatment for low potassium is relatively simple, and easier than for potassium excess. While monitoring her cardiac function in the ICU, Annie received multiple IV bags of potassium chloride in the hopes of quickly restoring her potassium balance. Her fluids were also aggressively replaced intravenously due to the significant dehydrating effect of the diuretics. Once I got her settled into the unit, I went home for the night and anticipated checking up on her early the following morning.

Overnight all was uneventful, and I received no pages about Annie or anyone else that I was following on the internal medicine teaching service. The following morning, I arrived at the hospital at 7:00 a.m. to complete my morning rounds. I was most interested in seeing how Annie was doing, so I began in the ICU. When I reviewed her labs on the computer, everything looked great—her potassium had rapidly normalized, sodium level improved, and her weight was up several pounds after multiple liters of IV fluids. All of her labs had been appropriately corrected and seemed to indicate a significant clinical improvement. Annie's overnight nurse had no concerning issues to report to me either. I optimistically made my way over to Annie's room, elated with her improvement and confident that I would encounter a happy, grateful patient showering me with richly deserved accolades.

Unfortunately, upon arriving at Annie's doorway, I didn't encounter any of the joyful emotions radiating from her that I had anticipated. In contrast, I found a frustrated and hostile patient.

"I hope that you're happy . . . Look what you doctors have done to me . . . My legs are awful, they positively look like elephant legs, tree trunks or whatever," she angrily vented to me. On examination, her legs showed no edema. *Does this woman have a distorted body image? Perhaps she struggled with anorexia or bulimia growing up as a teenager?*

"Annie, have you forgotten how yesterday went down?" I countered, staunchly refusing to back down from this bizarre confrontation. "You couldn't lift your head up off of a pillow because of life-threatening potassium and sodium depletion caused by *you* taking potent Mexican diuretics without a doctor's prescription!"

I was incredulous about this most peculiar emotional interaction. We had saved a woman from a potentially fatal metabolic condition, and not only was she ungrateful, she was enraged about the turn of events. The unexpected harsh criticism blindsided me in a situation where I expected to encounter an environment of appreciation.

"Well, I feel much better, so I just want to go home now!" she angrily responded. She then added a comment, dripping with sarcasm, "There is certainly nothing else you could be doing for me here right now."

I withstood a few more minutes of her assailing my character and competence before I politely excused myself. My internal anger felt out of sync with the ironic serenity of the quiet hallway. I brusquely leaned back against the wall, utilizing every fiber of my being to compose myself. I struggled to process what had just transpired between Annie and me. Our team had executed a medically sound, compassionately delivered treatment plan, and the seriously ill patient had positively recovered. But it was not enough for the patient, who remained adamantly dissatisfied. I was humbled to realize at that moment that another human being's frame of reference of health and happiness may be different from my own—perhaps even pathologic in tone.

A few minutes later I returned to Annie's room to review her medication list, discharge instructions and with a plan to follow up in the family medicine clinic in two weeks. She had softened her aggressive demeanor knowing of her impending departure to home. Our parting interaction was purely a robotic transaction, a simple exchange of only essential relevant medical information. As I left, I attempted a feeble smile and reminded her, "Please make sure that we see you back in the office in two weeks, it's very important."

"OK sounds good . . . I'll see you then," she replied in a noncommittal voice.

We never saw her again.

CHAPTER 10

DECEMBER

7:00 a.m. December 24, 1995. Obviously, Christmas Eve, but in the sphere of medical resident education, purely another day of in-house hospital call. At least that is what my fellow residents and I tried to tell ourselves. Driving in that morning to Waukesha Memorial Hospital, I attempted to minimize the special memories I would be missing: my wife's lasagna, Christmas carols, watching *It's a Wonderful Life*, culminating with a moving Midnight Mass at our local Catholic church. My wife and I were essentially newlyweds, with no children on the horizon. I cautioned my wife and immediate family that I would be quite busy and not to expect to hear from me through the day.

My December rotation was on Obstetrics, taking a complete 24-hour stint of call every three days. Call days were often hectic, typically having around five deliveries each day, along with countless patients to evaluate for labor, changes in fetal movement, urinary tract infections, preterm labor workups, and women coming in for medical induction of labor. Despite our resident team being entirely composed of family physicians, the obstetricians were incredibly supportive and were highly invested in our education and success. By month's end, I would participate in about fifty deliveries and upon completion of my training program, help bring around two hundred babies into the world. We were even the first surgical assistants on Cesarean sections, which was an invaluable clinical experience.

As I brought in my overnight bag to the doctor's lounge and changed into my scrubs, I looked out the window two floors down onto the sparsely populated parking lot. The weather was clear but cold, with temperatures in the mid-20s. The ground of the soccer field next door was covered in a faint alabaster patina of snow. It looked like we would have a white Christmas after all, but just barely. I glanced at the always-on TV in the lounge and saw an updated weather report: The local weatherman called for sunny skies the first part of the day, followed by more clouds and possibly one to three inches of snow. That was a mixed blessing—foul weather often caused a woman's water to break and to bring on labor, making my shift chaotic, but to me that was better than spending a 24-hour holiday shift inside, bored beyond imagination.

The perverse beauty of the 24-hour on-call shift on labor and delivery was always its pure unpredictable nature. You could be busy, bored, or have high stress/volumes in variable streaks throughout the day. As I traversed the corridor from our sleeping quarters to the birthing center (a new name back then), I had no prescient feeling about the upcoming flow of the day. After all, "It was Christmas, so people would rather be at home with their families," momentarily forgetting what service in the hospital I was working.

Upon arrival on the unit, I checked the whiteboard that contained the census of the expectant mothers on the service. The board was arranged like a grid, containing important info such as room number, patient initials, week of pregnancy, any pertinent medical information, and finally the critical nugget—the dilatation level of the cervix (0–10 cm, 10 cm fully dilated and ready for delivery), degree of softening (0–100%) and head position or station (ranged minus-3 to plus-3). A nearby computer screen displayed a laboring patient's contraction activity and fetal heart rate tracings. Only two patients were on the board, and they were not in active labor. It appeared they would be going home soon, and the board would be empty, at least for the time being. I took sign-out from the resident coming off of the 24-hour shift, and given the low census, the report was brief and to the point. At this juncture, things were shaping up for an uneventful day in the maternity world. We made a point to never utter the Q-word—"quiet"—which could be a jinx and result in an undesirable deluge of patients.

After getting settled and socializing with the nursing team for a few minutes, I set off to work. The two mothers-to-be and their husbands were very pleasant and comfortable. One had a few hours of contractions, but her cervix didn't dilate, so by definition she wasn't in labor. Her regular contractions had progressively diminished after a few hours of intravenous fluids, and I arranged to have her sent home. The other woman was concerned that her water broke. The telltale test for amniotic fluid is to complete a sterile speculum/pelvic exam, obtain a fluid sample, and examine it under the microscope. Amniotic fluid has sugars that cause the slide to crystallize, like frost on the windowpanes on the outside windows, a finding called "fern-ing." Her vaginal examination showed only minimal drainage and a closed cervix. The slide was negative for the characteristic branching pattern of amniotic fluid. Thus, mother-to-be #2 was also placed on the launchpad for discharge.

A couple of hours elapsed without incident, allowing me to read up on a couple of topics of interest in the obstetrics textbook. Late morning arrived, and I took the opportunity to head down to the cafeteria for an early lunch. In the residency world, we had a saying, "Eat when you can eat, sleep when you can sleep." Failing to take advantage of these windows of opportunity could result in a hungry, sleepless night.

As I gulped down my sandwich and chips, I glanced out the bay of south-facing windows and noticed a dramatic change—the brilliant sunny and cerulean skies were being inevitably replaced by ominous low-hanging, pewter-gray clouds, accompanied by some scattered early flurries. A uncomfortable flutter in my stomach made itself known. Perhaps this was a harbinger of not only meteorological change, but also an influx of mothers-to-be to the delivery unit. I efficiently finished my meal and scampered back up to the floor, uncertain of what I might encounter.

My gut instincts were proven correct. The unit clerk confirmed that three patients were already on their way into the hospital for possible onset of labor. Our typical protocol was to have the labor and delivery (L&D) nurse do a brief initial assessment. I would follow up with a short history and physical examination, and report my findings to the attending OB/GYN physician. All three patients arrived in short order, and while the nurses got acquainted with their expectant moms, I reviewed their office notes. Fortunately, all three of these young women had experienced uneventful pregnancies up to this point. In methodical succession, I introduced myself to the moms-to-be and their significant others, completed initial physical assessments and wrote my admission notes in the charts. All of the patients had two sensor belts attached to them: One transducer picked up the baby's heart rate while the other measured contractions of the uterus. To truly be in labor, a patient needed to have regular uterine contractions and changes in the cervix, the purse-string opening at the base of the uterus.

Normal labor and delivery is conventionally divided into three primary phases. Stage one begins with the onset of regular uterine contractions and ends with complete dilatation of the cervix (10 cm in diameter), which typically lasts up to twenty-four hours. The second stage begins with full cervical dilatation, active pushing and ends with delivery of the infant, usually around two to three hours. Finally, the third phase commences with delivery of the infant and ends with delivery of the placenta, a time span of twenty to thirty minutes. The true timing of these stages can be variable, with potential crises occurring at any time. I had several specific responsibilities as the resident physician on the obstetrics floor: perform initial evaluations on all admissions to L&D, make regular rounds at least every two hours on all laboring patients, respond rapidly to any urgent or emergent situations including precipitous delivery, and finally supporting the attending physicians and learning from them as much as possible.

Rebecca Winfield was a twenty-nine-year-old married woman, the first patient of the trio to arrive who seemed to be progressing the most rapidly in the labor process. By the mid-afternoon, her initial excitement about delivering her first child had dissipated, replaced by generalized discomfort and an emotional struggle with continual contractions of a uterus eager to be free of its beautiful bundle of joy. Subsequently, an epidural anesthesia had been placed, which helped to significantly alleviate her physical distress. Her contractions were effective and regular, and the baby's heart rate remained reassuring.

As the hours of the afternoon ticked away, the cervical numbers ticked up: 4, 6, 8, 9 cm, then completely dilated. I gave my attending, Dr. Mike Brennan, the heads-up at the 8 cm mark, and he made his well-timed appearance right as we began to prepare for some pushing. We prepped the surgical table and instruments for delivery and adjusted Rebecca's bed for the active process of coaxing the infant into the glories of the outside world. Every two or three minutes, the monitor's uterine bell curve and the slight creases and grimaces of Rebecca's forehead signaled the beginning of the contraction. She would take a deep cleansing breath, place her chin to her chest and "Push, push, push! 1, 2, 3, 4, 5, 6, 7, 8, 9, 10! and Again! Push, push, push!" sometimes followed by another count to ten until the contraction had subsided.

After about ninety minutes of this intermittent atypical aerobic workout, the baby's head began to descend low enough to separate the folds of the vaginal opening, labia majora and minora, a process referred to as crowning. This signaled that the delivery was a few contractions and minutes away. Dr. Brennan and I gowned and gloved up, preparing ourselves for another miracle of birth. With building anticipation, I attempted to strike a mental balance between the wonder and joy of the moment and maintaining the clinical focus to manage this critical stage of labor. I deftly arranged the instruments on the delivery table for organized convenience and ease of accessibility, a big crowd pleaser for my attending physicians. Doc Brennan and I had done several deliveries together already, so thankfully he was becoming quite comfortable with my level of confidence and skill set. He looked at me warmly, and his ice-blue eyes crinkled and sparkled above his surgical mask.

"OK Bruce, how 'bout you take the lead on this delivery? I'll be your assistant and be right beside you to lend a hand in case you need it, OK?"

"Sure Dr. Brennan, I appreciate that, thanks for the opportunity."

"No problem, let's work hard, I may try to get to the 5:00 p.m. Mass today."

At this point the vertex of the head emerged, rested and extended slightly past the vaginal opening. I palpated the suture lines of the skull to ascertain the presenting position of the infant's head. Left occiput anterior, i.e., facedown—that's a good sign, and should make for an easier delivery. I used a towel to support Rebecca's buttock area while her baby's head steadily and inevitably stretched and partitioned the final gateway to earthly existence.

"C'mon Rebecca! You can do it! Almost there!" I called out to her, sounding more like cheerleader and coach than obstetrician. After yet another salvo of standing ten counts, the baby's head broke free and was now completely outside on the mother's perineum. Thankfully, my support with the towel on the posterior side of the mother's vaginal area had prevented any significant tearing. Quickly, I checked around the baby's head for any umbilical cord wrapped around the neck. Not feeling any slimy tethering lasso, I utilized a little blue bulb suction device to clear the infant's mouth and then nose area of mucus secretions.

Next, I needed to ensure clear passage of the infant's shoulders, to verify there was no locking taking place, a complication called dystocia. Nope, nice adequate pelvic area. I gently cradled the baby's head and neck, lifting it carefully up toward the sky to prevent any unnecessary trauma and tearing to the mother's genital area. In a liquid motion, the remainder of the baby's body made a lightning-quick egress, followed by a paroxysmal parting cascade of clear, watery amniotic fluid. I deftly turned the infant around into my left arm and lap. I held the wondrous prize on my forearm, with the blessed head in the palm of my left hand. He looked beautiful and perfect. *A boy.* The parents had named him Charlie, and at that moment it seemed like the greatest name for a baby in the entire world.

"Congrats Rebecca! You have a beautiful baby boy! Nice job!" I called out, overwhelmed by birthing's pure joyous spectacle. I felt honored and privileged to be a part of it, let alone be a leading player in Charlie's arrival.

"Thanks Doc, thank you so much!" Rebecca and her husband replied in emotional and appreciative tones, swept away as well in the tremendous impact of the addition of a new life into this world. Even through Charlie's prominent wailing I could hear them quietly crying muted tears of happiness.

I placed two clamps on the umbilical cord, then handed the scissors to Mr. Winfield. "Would you like to cut the cord, Mr. Winfield?" I asked.

"Sure, I'd be honored," he replied, and in a deliriously happy and exhausted emotional fog proceeded to shakily divide and separate the now unnecessary umbilical lifeline. A few minutes later, a small expected gush of blood from the vaginal opening, a lengthening of the remnant of the umbilical cord, followed by the effortless and intact delivery of the placenta—stage three now completed, and just like that, the labor and delivery process drew to a glorious denouement.

Dr. Brennan looked at me bright-eyed, and I could tell by his eyes and tone of his voice that he was smiling. "Nice delivery there, Bruce. Should we inspect the perineum for any tears and stitch 'em up?"

"Sure," I replied. We inspected the vaginal area, and found two upper abrasions that did not need suturing, and one small laceration on posterior vaginal wall that required a few stitches and nothing else. After completing the surgical repair, I turned to look at the Winfields. They came in here as a dyad, a couple, and they would leave this hospital with one more new life, a family, a trio. I extended my congratulations once more, shook a grateful new father's hand, who unexpectedly offered, "Can we get a picture of the two doctors with baby Charlie?"

Two doctors. Humbly, I cradled baby Charlie once again, and along with Dr. Brennan completed our photo op. I gave Rebecca a heartfelt gentle hug before departing. The feeling was surreal, blessed and giddy, like I had had a couple of quick stiff drinks on a Friday night. As I sat in momentary contented reverie at the nurses' station, completing the requisite paperwork and delivery record, one of the labor and delivery nurses named Pamela quickly commanded my attention.

"Hey Dr. Rowe, Mrs. Anderson is complete and pushing right now. Dr. Harrison is on her way in. Can you come give us a hand?"

"You bet, no problem," I replied. Looks like the paperwork was going to wait awhile, no big loss, as it is never a favorite aspect for any doctor. Within the hour, Dr. Harrison and I completed the delivery process without any major issues. I returned to the front desk to find another OB nurse visibly needing assistance.

"Dr. Rowe, Room 5 is now getting ready to push, we need you!"

"OK—let's keep it going," I replied. As I got ready to enter that room I heard the unit clerk call out, "By the way, four more potentially laboring patients are on their way in now."

Another eighty minutes elapsed, and baby girl Isabella made her entrance into the world. Upon returning to the nurses' station and rechecking the whiteboard, all four of the laboring moms had arrived successfully. The monitors revealed that all of them were contracting, potentially indicating some degree of early labor. I reviewed all of the prenatal records for each patient, getting them tucked in and prepared for the delivery journey. Before I could complete hourly rounds on the new set of patients, another maternal delivery was imminent. One hour later, another baby girl, Lilly, was born without incident. The other three patients were laboring effectively and progressing more quickly than anyone on the team could have imagined.

I glanced out the window of one the patient rooms into the gathering inky darkness outside. The pinkish-yellow streetlights illuminated the gracefully falling snowflakes, with three inches of icy white meringue blanketing the vast expanse of the concrete parking lot. It confirmed my suspicions that it was going to be a crazy call night.

Throughout the night, a repetitive cycle continued unabated. Over the next few hours, several subsequent patients arrived on the L&D floor in early to active labor. It felt like Hercules and the Hydra; for every delivery I completed, seemingly two new pregnant ladies arrived to take her place. I kept up on the H&Ps, rounding and progress notes, but the delivery notes/summaries had to wait; too much important immediate doctoring needed to be completed. All night long, the amazing pace of arrival, labor, delivery and recovery continued. The number of deliveries that I racked up that day continued to accumulate: five, seven, ten, twelve deliveries and counting. A magical and unbelievable call session was eloquently unfolding on the night we celebrated the birth of the Christian Savior.

It was now 3:00 a.m. on Christmas Day, and the influx of incoming patients had finally slowed, although there were a still a few moms on the unit who were in the early stages of labor. I fought off the urge of complacency, cautiously aware that the last vestiges of the overnight could have a few remaining surprises.

Betsy waddled uncomfortably into the birthing center at around this time. Her face was creased with discomfort which clearly escalated every two to three minutes, then lasted about one minute before subsiding temporarily. The nurses and I quickly ushered her to a room. While they began an IV and hooked up the monitors, I introduced myself to Betsy and her husband. I completed a cervical check—she was already 5 cm dilated, a completely thinned-out cervix, and the baby's head was quite low. This was Betsy's second pregnancy, and these findings portended a rapid labor and delivery. Despite the early morning hour of the day, I paged Betsy's attending obstetrician, Dr. Nancy Sherwood, and briefed her on her laboring patient's status. She agreed that things could transpire quickly and made plans to come in within the hour unless something suddenly changed. Before trying to take a quick cat nap in the call room, I finished up some charting, then went to check on Betsy one last time.

Things had clearly changed over the course of the last thirty minutes. Betsy was animated, more uncomfortable. She had declined an epidural, and the IV pain medications were incompletely controlling her labor pains.

"Chips, Tom, dammitt!" she brusquely called out to her husband for some more ice chips.

"OK honey, comin' right up," a meek and cautious Tom replied.

I phoned Dr. Sherwood and notified her of the rapidly progressing labor; the cervix had opened to 8 cm, her contractions were almost one on top of the other, and the baby's head drew ever closer to the metaphysical gateway to the world. Dr. Sherwood said that she would come right away. Just then, I looked outside Betsy's hospital room window. It was now snowing heavily, with an unexpected six to nine inches of blowing, newly fallen snow. Unplowed roads, slippery stretches and poor visibility could make for a long drive in for a doctor from home. *I may be on my own for this delivery.*

Fifteen minutes later, Betsy was rapidly puffing and panting, and indicated a desire to push. Her follow-up vaginal check showed her to be completely dilated, the baby's head tantalizingly low in the birth canal. It was time to begin the active birthing process, yet my attending hadn't arrived yet. Unless completely unavoidable, it was considered bad form to deliver a baby without the senior physician present. Regardless of everyone's most conscientious efforts, it looked like the weather outside and the laboring mother inside were not going to cooperate with those plans.

Betsy was unhappy, but also very focused on the task at hand: get this baby delivered, and the seemingly unbearable pain will be gone. She yelled at Tom for more ice chips, sharply demanded from me how much longer until the baby would be delivered and when Dr. Sherwood would finally arrive. Her pain and frustration were understandable and palpable. I encouraged her to push as much as she needed, and if the infant came quickly, we were ready for it. On the monitor, the baby's heart rate looked good, so we were in no hurry to complete her delivery. However, the inevitable realities of the biology of the situation began to take over. This was going to my delivery all by my lonesome, something that I had never completed.

Within twenty minutes of the phone call to my senior obstetrician, baby Benjamin made a rapid appearance. He was another beautiful and healthy baby born that morning without complication, a Christmas morning blessing. I checked Betty's perineum for any tears or major injuries. A few small abrasions near the urethra, otherwise nothing that needed suturing. Dr. Sherwood arrived a few minutes later, apologizing for her tardiness generated by the storm. She was not angry with me for her having missed the delivery, but instead relieved that everything went according to plan. After reviewing the case, checking the baby and verifying nothing needed stitching, she quickly departed back for home. As her discomfort subsided, Betsy returned to a pleasant, warm baseline and made a point to thank me for my help with her delivery.

After everything was cleaned up, it ended up being six in the morning. I began to dictate Betsy's delivery note, only to find out after I completed it that I had fallen asleep and had no recollection of what I had said in the note. A couple of days later I had transcription pull that report for me to revise and review, certain that it was an unintelligible literary disaster. Much to my astonishment, the note was perfectly done—no blank spaces or inaccuracies related to my extreme level of exhaustion.

Christmas morning made a triumphant entrance, with a bright orange sunrise, clearing skies and a gentle icy breeze lightly swirling around the completed snowfall from overnight. Quickly I took stock of my inventory. Twenty-four hours, fourteen deliveries, a combined twenty-eight healthy moms and babies. I had only a half hour hour of rest all night, but paradoxically I felt refreshed and energized despite my sleep deprivation. It was a privilege to share in the birth experience with all of those families against the backdrop of the most celebrated birth in the Christian Era. I drove home post-call to begin the festivities of Christmas with my family, filled with a special sense of accomplishment, and grateful for the gift of being a family physician.

CHAPTER 11

SPILL

Practicing medicine can be a messy business . . . literally. On a regular basis, doctors are exposed to foul-smelling abscesses, uncontrolled bleeding, disgusting vomitus, and pungent stool. Malodorous substances spill out from patients, unexpectedly staining our clothes and assaulting our olfactory senses. My colleagues and I have always stoically accepted these noxious unsettling encounters as endemic to clinical medicine, even as they made their unwelcome appearances.

Wednesdays are a busy day in our office, with all of our providers diligently working a full midweek schedule. Most clinic days present challenges of difficult diagnoses and complex family dynamics, and often the "grocery list" of medical concerns to complete through the course of a fifteen- to twenty-minute appointment. Once in a great while, however, a day in the office can initially be deceptively uneventful. Those situations make me feel the most uneasy, because often karmic realignment will unexpectedly throw a curveball.

A clinic disaster of my own making shattered the placid office patient schedule many years ago. I had been in my practice at the Glendale Clinic for only a few months. The day had been moderately busy but nothing terribly exciting: a couple of young adults with viral bronchitis, a child with a painful ear infection, and a routine diabetic checkup in a very compliant individual. My next patient, Kenneth, worked as a laboratory technologist in our main hospital. He had been struggling with a painful ingrown toenail for the last several weeks. A variety of treatments, including antibiotic cream, warm-water soaks, and gingerly trimming the periphery of the nail area had failed to produce resolution. It was necessary to do a partial nail excision, in which one-third of the toenail is removed, the base is chemically cauterized, and the toenail grows back appropriately on its own.

I reviewed the treatment options with Kenneth. "In my training, this is the only way to get the ingrown toenail problem to definitively heal."

"Doesn't sound comfortable, but let's get it done today," he slowly agreed.

The technique for a partial nail excision is relatively straightforward. First, anesthesia consisting of a digital block injection is given at the base of the toe. Next, a hemostat or elevator is used to free up the stuck end of the nail, and then a blunt scissors cuts the affected nail away from the rest of the toenail. Finally, to prevent regrowth of the problematic toenail, a small Q-tip soaked in phenol is applied to obliterate the offending section of nail bed. I progressed through the procedure, removing the lateral nail without a hitch. All I needed was to apply the phenol treatment to complete the procedure.

I retrieved the phenol bottle from the medicinal cabinet and placed it on a silver tray. In the style of a waiter, I carried the bottle back down the clinical hallway. However, I needed to adjust my body position to get the exam room door reopened. This maneuver proved to be costly, as the bottle was heavier and had a higher-than-anticipated center of gravity. As I awkwardly moved back into Kenneth's room, the metal tray jerked, the fragile dark-glass bottle surged forward, sickeningly tumbled, and with an ominous sound shattered onto the tile floor. Immediately a distinctive organic aromatic odor filled the space.

Instantaneously it was apparent that this accident posed a significant problem. I moved Kenneth to another room, and my nurse quickly picked up the bigger pieces of glass and dabbed up the solution. Suddenly, the air became pungent, with my coworkers experiencing eye and respiratory irritation. With an escalating sense of panic regarding everyone's safety, I rushed to locate the Material Safety Data Sheet (MSDS), which listed all of the chemical information about phenol, including personal safety information and treatment recommendations for exposure. To my dismay, I couldn't find a listing for phenol in the first book I encountered. *How can that be?* I wondered. *Every chemical substance in the office needs to be accounted for in our manuals.*

While I was struggling with my quest to locate phenol's pertinent chemical information, our in-house pharmacist, Remy, came upon the scene. Remy was a kind Lebanese pharmacist who was intelligent, passionate, and would literally do anything for you. His knowledge of organic chemistry, unfortunately, was lacking. "It's an acid," he staunchly proclaimed, "we need to throw some bleach on it." Our staff, believing that a pharmacist would be secure in chemical principles, complied with his instructions and liberally doused the affected floor tile with the bleach compound.

Finally, after a few frantic minutes of searching, I located the phenol page in an alternative MSDS notebook. When I began reading, however, my heart sank—*Highly volatile, may be fatal if inhaled or with prolonged contact with the skin.* This had morphed into an industrial emergency and it was all my fault. I notified my clinic director and went back to the exam room to assess the situation. However, in transit I noticed the front desk area and patient waiting rooms now possessed the unmistakable odor of phenol. The bleach compound had reacted with the phenol solution and aerosolized it into an invisible toxic vapor. The fumes and exposures were spreading fast, and we needed to close the clinic and evacuate immediately. I notified all departments, closed all doors and orderly directed our entire staff to a safe region of the parking lot. I heard unsettling comments from my physician colleagues, grumbling, "I hope no one has any permanent injuries from this." They regarded me with unvarnished irritation that I had disrupted their busy clinic day.

Once everyone had left the building, the tableau was now set for further dramatic events. First, the fire department arrived, quickly followed by the hazardous materials team, and last but not least, the media, complete with cameras and on-site reporters. Mercifully, I was able to avoid the reporters' scrutiny as three of the nurses and I took an ambulance ride to our local emergency department. This was a necessary precaution due to the prolonged respiratory exposure to the toxic fumes. We were fortunate, as all of us had normal examinations and were able to be quickly discharged from the ER to home. Knowing that the safety and well-being of my coworkers was secured without any longstanding damage was reassuring.

A couple of hours later, I departed the ER and found my way back to the clinic at around 2:00 p.m. after the all-clear was given to reenter the building. What normally should have been a bustling clinic now took on the eerie unnerving appearance of a post-apocalyptic ghost town. All of the interior doors were propped open, and large circulatory fans blasted pressurized air throughout the facility. A faint odor of the organic phenol still lingered everywhere, a poignant reminder of how my momentary clumsiness shut down an economically vibrant clinic for an entire business day. Mindlessly I gathered up some charts and paperwork, and unceremoniously left the office for home. As I walked out the front door, a skeleton crew of front office staff was congregating for an impromptu conference. They glanced at me seriously, then returned to each other. They spoke in whispers, but I clearly overheard an ominous comment: "Somebody could lose their job over this."

Oh brother! That certainly wasn't a contingency I had thought about at this point. *Could they really follow through on something like that?* Of course, no one is indispensable in a health system workplace, and that would also include physicians. However, the termination of a physician was usually related to instances of grossly inappropriate and unprofessional conduct. After thoughtful consideration I reasonably concluded that even as a young physician, this type of disciplinary action was not justified. Still, the prospect of not being in the good graces of my partners and clinic team bothered me as I contemplated the atmosphere awaiting me in the office the next morning.

My temporary gloominess that evening was interrupted by an optimistic epiphany: When encountering a difficult situation, I could either sit idly by as a helpless spectator or take positive corrective action. It was time for me to exercise affirmative control. In the back of my home closet I located my Disney World Goofy hat. At our local grocery store I purchased a large bag of Butterfinger mini-sized candy bars, aptly named for the circumstances. As I wore my crazy chapeau the next morning and passed out my sugary treats to my coworkers, I could see their tension and resentment steadily dissipate.

For years thereafter staff members on a warm sunny day would jokingly inquire, "Hey Dr. Rowe, how 'bout we have a chemical spill today?" I realized that people can be defined by not only by achievements but also displaying grace and humility during embarrassing situations. Crazy days like these often create powerful reflections, as well as lighthearted moments of laughter.

Spills are not confined to unanticipated patient odors or fluid. An elderly patient who takes an unforeseen tumble is a distressing spill event of its own, often resulting in a loss of independence. Marvin was a warm, bear-like man whose active lifestyle belied his chronological age of eighty-four years young. He and his wife traveled all over the country in their medium-sized RV, enjoying every minute of their epic journeys. At his semiannual visits in our office, he regaled me with stories of trips to breathtaking panoramic Western scenes and rocky windswept ocean coasts.

He arrived for a visit at an unusual time of year on his travel calendar, interrupting his typical spring break excursion. I watched him gingerly walk in with an atypically unsteady gait. Marv looked weak, fatigued and certainly not himself.

"Hi ya Marv, looks like you've not been enjoying your vacation," I began.

"That's the truth," he replied. "I got up off of a picnic bench at our resort in Florida, stumbled and lost my footing. It was a hell of a tumble. Ever since then I feel weak all over."

"Sounds weird to me. Any problems with losing control of your bowels or your bladder?"

"I don't know. It seems like I have to rush to the bathroom to pee all of a sudden, although I can't get there very quickly. I've never experienced anything like this."

"Any other weird symptoms like fevers, chills, rashes, chest pain, shortness of breath, night sweats or fainting episodes?"

"No—none of those things, just feel like I have no strength in any muscle of my body."

Marvin typically was very stoic and didn't complain much, which only served to intensify my concerns. *Generalized weakness? Is he having a stroke? Guillain-Barre Syndrome? Subdural hematoma? Conversion disorder?* All of these scenarios seemed less likely. His physical exam revealed an impressive neurologic examination: generalized body weakness, and diminished deep tendon reflexes throughout. He had no fever, recent immunizations or viral infections, so Guillain-Barre Syndrome seemed doubtful. His findings were most consistent with cervical myelopathy, which is a herniated disc of the upper spine causing serious compression of the spinal cord. It is an urgent

151

neurosurgical issue that if not rapidly addressed could lead to quadriplegia. Marv's cervical spine X-ray showed a shifting of the second and third cervical vertebrae which indeed could cause cord impingement. Subsequently, Marv was urgently hospitalized, and an MRI of the cervical spine confirmed a high-level herniated cervical disc with significant spinal cord compression. The following day he underwent cervical spine decompression with fixation of the vertebrae without complications. Fortunately he made a full recovery with return of his strength and coordination.

Accidents and injuries always hit home when your immediate family is acutely affected. Mom called me at university unexpectedly on an Easter Sunday evening, and sadly told me that Grandma Helen was in the hospital, having fallen and fractured her right hip. She proceeded through the total hip replacement procedure without any significant difficulties. After her mild postoperative confusion resolved, I drove home to pay her a visit. My grandma had been in our county hospital innumerable times for a multitude of medical ailments and surgeries, so there was a sense of routine with her once again residing in a hospital bed. When I came into her room, the noontime sun poured in through her large windows, with an expectant springtime hope for healing.

"Hi ya, Grandma," I quipped happily and relieved. "How're you feeling today? How's the dinner menu here?"

"Ah, it's OK here I guess . . . the food is tolerable, the pain meds and therapy seem to be working reasonably well, and I hope to get the hell out of here real soon." I was relieved at the return of her baseline cantankerous behavior.

"I was so sad to hear about your hip, are you going to rehab for a while?" I delicately asked.

"Yes, your mother thinks rehab would help my hip heal, move better and make the pain go away. Guess I'll go along with the plan for now."

"I sure hope it's not too long, Grandma."

"I'll do what it takes to make it a short stay," she responded with a not-so-subtle twinge of her trademark grit and determination.

We spent a couple of hours visiting together, sharing updates with each other about our lives, and the ubiquitous small-town local gossip. Soon the afternoon began to wind down, and it was time to for me to head back to the university. I gave her a hug and a kiss goodbye, and as I walked toward the door she issued her friendly reminder:

"Make sure you drive over by my hospital window so I can wave bye-bye to you."

This was a tradition that dated back to when I was a young boy. At that time, children under fourteen were prohibited from seeing people on the inpatient floors. Thus, I was not able to physically visit my grandmother during her previous hospital stays. My parents would have Grandma Helen give a friendly wave down to me on the street from her hospital room window so that I would see that she was happy and healing.

I walked out of the hospital, and upon reaching the parking lot turned and looked back and upward at the spartan white brick edifice. I carefully counted over the number of windows over to Grandma's hospital room. It was then that I saw her, cloaked in her royal blue robe, radiant smile, the fluorescent lighting in the background illuminating the outlines of her silver-gray hair, as a Madonna. I felt a rekindling of those same childhood reassurances identifying Grandma's luminous appearance framed by the simple rectangular hospital window. We exchanged hearty waves and appreciative smiles, then I revved up my old Chevy for the return journey to Iowa City. I felt the warm salty tears of happiness spill down my cheeks as I reveled in the unspoken spiritual connection between the two of us.

Arriving back at my beloved U of I, in passing I glanced up at the sparkling, towering alabaster wings of the University Hospital. The expansive bank of patient room windows were of reflective glass, impervious to inward viewing from passersby. I contemplated the grandmothers and other patients in those rooms, battling their challenging respective illnesses. Later, as a medical student within those walls, I strived to educate patients and facilitate the emotional healing connections between clinicians, patients and families.

Early childhood for me was a lot of fun, in that being the firstborn child in a family afforded a tremendous number of advantages. Typically first time parents are generally younger and more energetic, not dividing their time and attention among multiple children. I was the sole beneficiary of my mother's and father's love and devotion until I was a second grader. However, as I grew older, I noticed that many of my friends had younger and older siblings. I craved the company of another young person in my family with whom to play games, quarrel, and even physically wrestle. My desire for a younger sibling became so strong that I once mistakenly proclaimed to the neighborhood that I was going to be a big brother, a rumor emphatically quashed by my parents. As a teenager, I belatedly learned that my mom and dad had attempted conceiving a second child multiple times, but had issues with infertility and multiple miscarriages.

Finally in the late summer of 1975, success! My parents proudly announced that my mother was with child and had surpassed the hazards of the first trimester of pregnancy. For months, with excitement I awaited the arrival of my sibling, witnessing my mother's protuberant belly, feeling the lightning-quick kicks beneath my small hands. It felt like the greatest Christmas present ever awaiting its momentous earthly arrival. As the winter prepared to give way to springtime, in February of 1976 my little sister Monica Lynn made a beautiful yet medically uneventful appearance.

Having a kid sister in my life was a break from the previous monotony of just my parents and me spending time together. Here I had a front-row seat watching this little newborn grow and develop into an infant, a toddler, and a little girl. My parents showed me how babies spoke, moved and interacted with the world. Our house which had been dominated by toy cars, trains, blocks and GI Joes gave way to pink and purple clothes and colors, baby dolls who could wet themselves, Easy Bake Ovens, and pretend kitchen sets. We played silly games and roamed the neighborhood together. She had her own distinctive personal gifts, quirks and tastes.

Even though we were nearly eight years apart in age, we still maintained a bewildering ability to aggressively play and fight together, much to the consternation of my parents and maternal grandmother. It was in this seemingly undramatic Midwestern setting that my world appeared to collapse on me one cool February evening.

Monica and I were on the living floor playfully wrestling with each other as usual. She had just recovered from a classic winter cold a couple of weeks ago. I was eleven years old, my sister had just turned four. In the process of rolling around on the floor, my elbow inadvertently caught my sister on the nose. It was an accident, and it didn't appear to contact her face very intensely. She didn't even cry out, get angry, or indicate anything was amiss. However, within a few seconds, the aftermath of the innocuous collision was mortifying. She began to bleed profusely from her nose, and this was no ordinary case of nosebleed. Like a poorly attended spigot, the crimson fluid upwelled from her nose and began to spill out onto the carpet. I grabbed Monica and rushed her to the kitchen.

"Help somebody! Somethin' happened to Monica and she's bleedin' real bad!" I called out indirectly to any parental unit within shouting distance.

My dad sprinted into the kitchen first. "What the hell?" he exclaimed in a vitriolic mixture of surprise and rising anger.

"We were wrestling on the floor and I bumped her nose and it just started bleeding, it was an accident . . ." I trailed off meekly. *What just happened?* I thought to myself in a panicked, horrified state of internal tribulation. I had never intentionally, or even accidentally hurt anyone previously in my lifetime. *What's wrong with me?*

I quickly became aware of the ominous and emergent nature of the hemorrhage. My mom appeared a split second later, and her visible fear and sadness upon seeing her injured daughter sent peals of shame radiating through my psyche. "Bruce! How could you do this? I can't believe that you deliberately hurt your baby sister! You don't even know your own strength, you can't control yourself!" Her chain of accusations exhibited growing terror mixed with simmering rage at my perceived actions.

By this time my father's naval medic training had engaged, and his actions were swift and decisive. With militaristic precision he laid my sister down on the kitchen table, applying steady squeezing pressure to my sister's nostrils in a fervent hope of quelling the bleeding. I was stunned at the relentless egress of bloody fluid emanating from the nostrils. Many times on the playground, I had witnessed more than my fair share of scrapes, bumps and nosebleeds. This bleeding process was much more dramatic, both in terms of the rate and volume involved. I visibly and subconsciously sensed the icy stares of anger and indignation from my parents as they struggled to stabilize my sister's blood loss. After thirty-five harrowing minutes, the nosebleed relinquished its life-threatening scarlet torrent. My mother spoke with our family doctor, Dr. Graham, who wanted to see Monica first thing the following morning.

I went to bed that night feeling like a criminal outcast for the first time. My mom in a tired voice simply stated, "Get to bed. We'll talk about this more in the morning." With a sense of shame and dejection, I changed into my pajamas and unceremoniously climbed into bed. I laid awake, restless and sniffling silently to myself in the cold, inhospitable darkness of my bedroom. An unrelenting sense of personal disappointment and fear of the next day's impending consequences encompassed me. It felt like the overwhelming clouded winter chill outside of my bedroom window. *Am I turning into a mean and violent person?* Certainly, things would correct themselves overnight and the world would be set aright again come tomorrow morning.

Alas, relief from my tribulations did not come with the breaking of the dawn. I was greeted to an awkward emotional distance from my parents at breakfast and experienced a red-hot sense of guilt for apparently having inflicted physical harm upon my sister. My mom drove me to school that morning in a profound enveloping milieu of silence and anger. Monica rode along in the front seat, prepared for her visit to the doctor. Shortly before I departed the car for school, my mom spoke to me in an angry, unsympathetic tone that I had never experienced from her:

"You need to think long and hard about what you did to your sister yesterday. What kind of monster does this to his kid sister who worships the ground that he walks on? Why look at all of these bruises that you gave her!" Mom lifted up Monica' shirt to reveal multiple small irregular oblong purple violaceous spots diffusely scattered throughout her trunk, torso and extremities. In retrospect, I now realize that they were petechiae not caused by physical abuse, but at age eleven, I did not have this medical insight. I certainly wasn't stupid enough to challenge a grown-up, especially my mother.

"Mom, I swear I only lightly bumped her nose . . . I didn't hit her anywhere else . . . it was an accident . . ." In vain I weakly tried to defend myself. No one believed me, and my sister was too young and scared to help plead my case. Glumly, I exited the car and began the long painful walk up toward the schoolhouse door. *I love my sister and I'm not a monster . . . at least I don't think that I am . . . maybe my parents are right about me . . . I guess that I am becoming a bad person.*

Mom gave me a serious, furtive parting glance, devoid of hugs or a peck on the cheek. "I'll take Monica to the doctor this morning, and after we find out what's going on, your father and I will discuss your punishment over dinner later tonight." Her voice and delivery were cold, cutting and undiplomatic.

"OK," I numbly acknowledged my adverse verdict and trudged off to school. I said a quick prayer for my sister and myself that morning and tried to muddle through all of my studies that day. Once school dismissed, I walked over to Grandma Helen's house to wait for further word on Monica's condition, emotionally preparing myself for the sentencing which would be meted out later that evening.

When I arrived at Grandma's house, I was astonished to find that my mom and sister were still at the doctor's office. "Dr. Graham thinks that your sister has a disease called Shone-Henox," Grandma informed me. "They are running some more tests now." In retrospect, she actually meant Henoch-Schonlein purpura, a common vasculitis which could present in this fashion. *Could it be that the nosebleed and bruising was a medical problem and not my fault after all?*

At that very moment in Dr. Graham's office, events were unfolding that portended my medical vindication: The bleeding event was related to a new-onset hematological condition, and not related to the careless actions of an older sibling. A bleeding time test was completed by poking my sister's ear, and normal clotting time was about seven minutes. Monica's bleeding time was an astronomical twenty-seven minutes. A follow-up complete blood count (CBC) confirmed a diagnosis and found an explanation for the horrific nosebleed. Her platelet count was only 12,000—normal levels are typically around 150-400 thousand. Platelets are absolutely essential for controlling bleeding, and Monica only had 10 percent of the normal desired platelet count. She had a critically low platelet level and would now need to be hospitalized. However, my hometown medical center had no pediatricians, so my sister was transferred to the larger town in the next county, Ottumwa, to see the pediatrician, Dr. Mark Levinthal.

Upon her arrival on the pediatric ward, literally a marathon twenty-six miles away, the correct medical diagnosis was finally rendered: Idiopathic Thrombocytopenic Purpura (ITP), caused by antibodies against platelets generated by my sister's recent viral infection. ITP patients can chew up platelets at an alarming rate, and in some circumstances drop the platelet counts down to serious, life-threatening levels.

Upon admission to the hospital, Monica was placed in a bed with extra padding to prevent further bleeding and trauma, and then her treatment was initiated: simply, immunosuppression with corticosteroids, medium- to high-dose prednisone tapered over a period of a few weeks. The response and recovery was definitive and rapid: Her platelets hit 45,000 on day one, 175,000 on day two, culminating at 325,000 on the third day, a day for discharge back to home. On the final day in the hospital, Dr. Levinthal allowed me into Monica's room while he made his morning rounds, and helped complete my absolution and vindication process.

"Luckily Bruce and Monica picked the right day for a wrestling match, so that we were able to witness a significant bleeding event. Had she dropped her platelet count any lower, she could have been at risk for a catastrophic cerebral hemorrhage or other life-threatening bleeding." Dr. Levinthal's kind face and warm delivery of good news was the perfect balm for my raw emotional wounds.

My parents' faces seemed to abruptly soften toward me in the wake of that profound medical observation from the pediatrician who saved my sister's life. I was too incapacitated by weighty emotional relief from the turn of events to smile, hug him or break into sobs. As I allowed those words to sink in, I became overjoyed by my sister's recovery. *I still had my sister with me and she was going to live!* The spills of blood and negative familial emotions from those last several days had officially evaporated, and our family could move forward. Looking back, I fondly realized that not only a doctor could heal a patient, but also repair the breach between a son and his parents.

It was 3:30 a.m. on a chilly, snowy Sunday January morning when my pager abruptly came to life, its obnoxious warbling demanding attention. I groggily turned onto my side, squinted at the readout and called the answering service. Subsequently, I was connected to the residence of Mrs. Bennett, the preacher's wife who was due any day now with her first baby.

"Hi Dr. Rowe, it's Suzanne Bennett . . . my water broke about thirty minutes ago, and I have been having contractions every five minutes. Should I go into the hospital?"

"Yes Suzanne, that sounds reasonable," I replied, now more awake and on secure mental footing. "I will meet you there in a little while."

"OK, thanks, Doctor," the phone call terminated. I laid awake in bed for about a half an hour, fighting the siren song of a warm bed, comfy pillow and my wife's cuddling embrace. My obstetrical experience and intuition with similar situations told me that this labor may progress a little quicker than expected. I hopped into the shower to quickly clean up, and as I stepped out my home phone rang—it was Labor and Delivery at the downtown hospital.

"Hi Dr. Rowe, it's Candace, I'm taking care of Ms. Bennett here. I know that it's hard to believe, but she is nearly completely dilated and feels like pushing."

Shit, I misjudged it . . . I shoulda skipped the shower. "OK," I tried to feign a sense of nonchalance, "I will be there in fifteen minutes." I threw on an old green oxford button-down shirt and khakis to convey a sense of professional attire, then dashed out the door. A frigid, chilled winter wind greeted me, and four inches of newly fallen snow covered the roads. I hit 85 miles per hour on the freeway during my frenetic quest to arrive at the hospital in time. Mentally I crossed my fingers not to incur the wrath of a highway patrolman nor lose control on the incompletely plowed roadway. Fortunately, I pulled into the doctor's parking lot exactly a quarter hour later, and sprinted up to the labor and delivery suite.

Breathlessly I entered Suzanne's room, and while she had not delivered yet, the look on her face and contraction pattern indicated that the newborn's arrival was imminent. There was no time to change—I was going to need to literally roll up my sleeves, gown up and get to work. I completed a vaginal check—the infant's head was positioned right outside the vaginal opening, and externally appeared with each contraction, a phenomenon known as crowning. A few pushes ensued, and seemingly smoothly and effortlessly, the Bennett's baby was born. A beautiful baby girl, *Hannah.*

"Congrats guys—she's adorable!" I inspected the vaginal area for any lacerations that need stitching. Thanks to Suzanne's control and self-discipline during the critical pushing phase of delivery, nothing needed to be repaired. "Sorry that I timed it so late, I thought that I would have had a few more minutes."

"Wouldn't have wanted you to miss it, Doc," a tired Suzanne replied with a surprising degree of warmth.

"Oh boy, I was supposed to preach this morning too!" Reverend Bennett chimed in.

I laughed at his impish remark. "I think you have a valid excuse today."

He smiled in that special manner that I have seen on the faces of countless new fathers. "Yeah, I guess the congregation will understand, I'm sure I can find a substitute."

The delivery process completed, I thanked the Bennetts for the privilege of the delivery and proceeded to head for home. Hopefully I could get in a few more hours of sleep, but the lingering emotional high of bringing a new little one into the world would be difficult to suppress. As I was getting undressed and back into my pajamas for some rest, I suddenly discovered it—a sizable amoeba-like patch of a blood stain from the delivery on the cuff of my right shirt sleeve. It must have leaked under my gown onto the fabric. My initial response was *Oh crap, my wife is going to kill me!* but moments later, I realized my latest spill was a badge of honor. It was a symbol of Hannah's delivery, a special shared parental moment, and like a pen placed to paper, an indelible mark of the joys of being a family doctor.

I now realize that medicine is not a neat and orderly process, but rather a constant battle with forces of physical disease, social chaos and emotional disorder. Whether caused by an accident, bleeding or a joyous delivery, unforeseen circumstances can be stressful, unsettling, or even a pleasant surprise. The inexorable entropy of life can be distressing and discouraging if I purely focus on the immediate spills of blood, trauma and emotional desperation. The critical piece in these circumstances is for me to remain optimistic and calm, allowing my self-confidence and expertise to rectify damage and promote an atmosphere of healing.

CHAPTER 12

BRONZED

Bronze is an elemental alloy which has been a critical and ubiquitous metallic component in human existence for thousands of years. In elegant statuary, civilizations through the centuries have immortalized their heroes and commemorated important battles. The Bronze Age propelled mankind to a new technological level with improved tools and, unfortunately, more-sophisticated weapons. Despite taking a back seat to gold and silver, an Olympic bronze medal is a very high honor and signifies an athlete "has reached the podium." Stronger than wood or fiber, more workable than stone, this dark-brown amalgam has proven to be critical in many practical applications. These warm chestnut shades occasionally show up in medical practice in unusual situations and in daily living, conjuring up many important and treasured memories.

Karen was a pleasant mother and grandmother who had been a patient of mine for many years. She and her sister founded their own small company in town and had developed it into an economically strong enterprise. At her appointments we would chat about her family and her business, but most importantly, we exchanged stories about our golf games and gave each other tips. Karen enjoyed playing golf all year round; in fact, she usually took a few weeks off during the winter months to hone her game in South Florida. During our office encounters, I offered some insights into her driving off the tee, and she would suggest ways to improve my lousy short-game approach to the green. Outside of an unfortunate diagnosis of breast cancer that was quickly identified, effectively treated and placed into remission, she had generally been fairly healthy, with the exception of a unique recent medical issue.

An early sign of medical trouble surfaced a couple of years into our clinical relationship together. She had been gaining weight more readily over the winter months, not losing it again in the spring and summer, and feeling more fatigued as the day wore on. Subsequently, she developed issues with dry, itchy skin, and her hairstylist noted that her hair was falling out more easily. At a recent office visit, I noticed that the outer third of her eyebrows seemed to fade away into nothing—Karen denied grooming this area. Finally, I examined her thyroid gland and it felt diffusely enlarged, not markedly so like a goiter, no concerning nodules, but abnormal nonetheless.

A quick and simple blood test showed that her thyroid-stimulating hormone level (TSH) was elevated, which was diagnostic of underactive thyroid disease, also known as hypothyroidism. Hypothyroid patients have a deficiency of thyroid hormone levels, and as a result struggle with fatigue and all the physical ailments that Karen was reporting. A simple treatment with prescription thyroid hormone supplement was helpful—her weight declined back to her baseline, her energy level improved, and the other skin and hair problems that were bothering her completely resolved. She and I were thrilled that her quality of life quickly reverted back to normal. Her endocrine problems appeared to have resolved, and she was ready for another enjoyable season out on the links.

I began to notice something unusual about Karen when she returned from her Florida trip the following spring. She had developed quite a pronounced bronze tan to her skin during her winter sojourn down South, which seemed plausible, given the amount of time she spent outside under the bright ultraviolet rays of the sun. However, as spring wore on, she continued to maintain near-mahogany hue, despite no trips to exotic tropical locales and a relatively cloudy March and April in Milwaukee that year. At her six-month thyroid gland check in early May, she seemed to shrug it off and not give it much thought.

"I guess that I tan much easier than most people and hang on to the color for a long time," she contemplated thoughtfully.

Her acceptance of the peculiar situation provided me with some comfort, but that was short-lived. When I checked her lab studies that day, her thyroid function was normal, but there was an unexpected finding: Her sodium level was decreasing, while her potassium level began to climb and was moving out of the normal range. I reviewed her medication list for any unusual compounds, diuretics, supplements or any recent changes to her regimen—nothing seemed out of the ordinary. Because her physical exam was unremarkable other than her grandiose tan, we planned to recheck her labs in about two weeks. When we reconvened in a fortnight, her labs only looked worse, with the gap between the sodium and potassium levels growing ever wider. It was an unusual, confounding problem with an unclear source; regardless of the etiology, it was rapidly requiring attention.

OK Bruce, let's think—what would cause a sudden change in her metabolic studies like that? Low aldosterone? Secretly using diuretics for weight loss? But the bronzed skin which has persisted for weeks . . . that sounds like what John F. Kennedy had in his prime, adrenal failure or specifically, Addison's disease. She has never been on long-term corticosteroids such as prednisone though—could this be primary adrenal failure? It seemed like a long shot, but it would explain all of her lab and exam findings.

I arranged for Karen to complete a test at the hospital, where she would be given an injection of an adrenal gland-stimulating hormone, and then checking her cortisol levels at baseline, then thirty and sixty minutes later. A normal test would show the cortisol levels rising with each of the three checks. In Karen's case, that didn't happen; in fact, her cortisol fell over the sixty minutes of testing, which was positive for adrenal insufficiency. This particular situation was not caused by excessively prescribed corticosteroids from the medical community; rather, this most likely was the result of an autoimmune condition. I consulted my endocrine specialist about my case of primary Addison's disease. Karen was started on prednisone and a secondary medication, a mineralocorticoid called fludrocortisone, to help her hold on to her sodium and excrete her potassium. Over a period of weeks her electrolytes normalized, and the prominence of her brawny tan steadily decreased. I was gratified to see her quickly responding to our interventions.

Endocrinology, the study of specialized glands, their hormones and their effects on the metabolism of the body, can be challenging for me. My personality, training and background in engineering coupled with my tendency to visualize concepts works well with beating hearts, breathing lungs and physiologic processes, but not so much with ethereal concepts like hormones, electrolytes or kidneys. If I remain open to complex modes of thinking outside of my intellectual comfort zone, I can ultimately arrive at the correct diagnosis and help my patient.

Father Frank Castelli was a retired Catholic priest, who spent his winter months shepherding a parish in Miami, Florida, and the rest of the year filling in for vacationing priests here in Milwaukee. We had seen him through a few harrowing hospitalizations for heart failure, and now in his early eighties he had begun to slow down a bit. I enjoyed our visits because of his thoughtful insight, interesting activities and engaging personality.

One day the discussion turned to a topic that he truly loved—playing golf. He had been a fair-to-middling golfer in his younger days, with a handicap in the low teens. Fondly, he recalled playing in the local Italian-American golf outing, and how he enjoyed reacquainting himself with many of his friends with a shared cultural heritage. As he spoke, his already kind and happy gray eyes took on an even livelier appearance, almost a pure manifestation of joy. Frank was not as strong as he had been, but still moved reasonably well, which gave me an idea.

"Frank, how about you and me go out and play nine holes of golf and grab dinner next week?"

"Really? You'd take me golfing? Just so ya know, I can't hit the ball very far nor play very fast anymore . . ." He was brimming with excitement and flashed a broad toothy grin.

"Sure, while you are hitting your balls it will buy me time to go searching in the woods for all of my sliced golf balls," I replied, tongue firmly in cheek. "How about next Tuesday, it's my afternoon off."

"Yes, I'm free, see you then!"

The following Tuesday was a pleasantly warm early June day, a perfect time to hit the links. I picked up Frank and drove over to one of our municipal courses, which the gentle spring rains had turned into a verdant carpet of lush Kentucky bluegrass. A gentle easterly wind brought a slight cool breeze off of nearby Lake Michigan, enough to suppress the heat and humidity, yet not leave us chilled. Upon renting a cart, securing our bags, and making sure that Frank was properly situated, we took off for the first tee box.

Frank's first tee shot hugged close to the ground, and only traveled about seventy-five yards, but it was straight, which was more than I could say about my high-arching slicing first stroke. After I dropped Frank off at his ball I located my ball, which by this point had caromed completely into the adjacent fairway. As I began to address my ball in preparation for my second shot, I snuck a glance over at Frank in the proper first fairway. He was happily sauntering up the short green grass, hitting the ball multiple times, all tight to the ground, going for minuscule distance, but consistent and straight nonetheless. I eventually corrected my ball into the right fairway, and soon Frank and I were approaching the first green in the cart together. As we were getting ready to chip our balls onto the green, he turned to me with a deep sense of gratitude and said, "Thanks so much, Bruce, for doing this for me, I haven't played golf in a long time and this means so much."

"You're welcome, Frank, I'm having a great time, glad that you're still able to play in your eighties."

The remainder of the round essentially was a reenactment of the first hole. Frank's choppy, pugilistic strokes went straight up the fairway, a staccato counterpoint to my dramatic, inaccurate shots back and forth down the course's corridors. After a little over two hours, we putted our final balls on the ninth green. The summer sun was beginning to make its daily downward trek toward the lush tree line at the edge of the golf course, and cast its slanted warm summer rays directly upon us. As I waited my turn to putt I looked at Frank, and in my mind saw him as he was forty years ago: a young attractive priest, his unmistakable Romanesque look with olive bronzed skin, jet-black hair, erect posture, in stark contrast to his current hunchbacked appearance. He putted the ball from ten feet with an air of confidence that was a throwback to his earlier days of golfing excellence, and we cheered as it entered the cup dead center with perfect speed and rotation. My putt rimmed out for another inevitable three-putt, and after shaking hands, we grabbed dinner at his favorite Greek restaurant. After a relaxing and enjoyable meal I dropped Frank off at his apartment, and then I turned and headed for home.

Later on that pleasant summer evening, as I savored a beer on my back patio, I contemplated the day's events. I never thought playing a round a golf and socializing with an eighty-year-old man could be so enjoyable.

A couple of weeks later, I received a thank-you note from Frank. It was a beautiful small card, with a Madonna and child icon of the cover. Inside it read:

Dear Bruce,

Thanks for the great golf, nice weather, your company and wonderful dinner last Tuesday. I had such a fantastic time and will treasure it always. But most importantly, thanks for thinking of me and spending your Tuesday afternoon with me for a few hours. Never lose your kind and healing spirit, it has served you well.

In gratitude,
Frank

Over the succeeding years, Frank and I saw each other often, both in the doctor's office and socially when he ultimately moved over to the retirement community to live out his final years. His heart failure and other chronic conditions progressively wore him down until he peacefully succumbed to the medical insults a few years later while in hospice care. I fondly recall how happy Frank looked on the last green of the golf course, interlaced within the lengthening shadows of the tall oak trees and the deep alloyed orange-red glow of the setting copper sun.

A few years ago, as I approached my fortieth birthday, I came to a painful realization that I had not completed many items on my ubiquitous bucket list. As a loyal, born and bred Hawkeye, I had always wanted to participate in the annual Iowa statewide bicycle trek called RAGBRAI. It is an acronym for Register's Annual Great Bicycle Ride Across Iowa, put on by the *Des Moines Register* newspaper every year on the last full week in July. Every year, about 12,500 bicyclists begin on a Sunday at the Missouri River on the western edge of the state, then over a seven-day period traverse the towns and countrysides of Iowa, finishing ultimately at the Mighty Mississippi River on a Saturday afternoon, triumphantly dipping their front bicycle tire in its muddy, meandering waters. Every year a variable route ensures that different parts of the state appreciate the awesome spectacle of cycling humanity. For one week, the rest of the country and world get to experience the small-town hospitality and the "Iowa nice" attitude of the local people, which has been a source of personal pride.

The thought of pedaling five hundred-plus miles in a week across rural, often rolling and hilly terrain in almost any permutation of weather felt a little daunting to me, as a busy medical practice had made me a little bit flabby around the middle. I seized this moment to encourage myself to get back into shape and accomplish a unique fitness goal. Finally the ice, snow and bitter chill of winter subsided, and the warmer temperatures and longer spring days made their entrances into southeastern Wisconsin, and none too early.

I began preparing for RAGBRAI in late April, with multiple long training rides out into the countryside. Riding through town, I turned northward onto an abandoned, paved old railroad trail, then moved westward out of the city. The beautiful homes of my suburb gave way to rolling hills, russet-brown stubbly cornfields, and pastures of grazing cows and horses. Dairy farms with their large milking barns and deep coffee-colored silos capped with silvery domes popped up on the landscape, with occasional small clusters of forests dotting the view. Alongside the road ran a rail line, frequented by short-length trains consisting of single locomotives towing a few oxide-red boxcars. A slightly brisk, stiff westerly wind greeted me as I pushed into the countryside.

Farther west were some steeper hills and climbs, topped with large oaks and maples, and an occasional rural Lutheran or Catholic church. These hills represented the residuals of the Wisconsin glaciation of the last Ice Age, which deposited large dome-shaped landforms which the locals referred to as the Kettle Moraine. The spectacular views provided some distraction for me with my excessively labored respirations and rapidly tiring bicycling legs. Downhills were exhilarating and I attempted to enjoy them as long as I could, and utilized their momentum for the inevitable uphill to follow.

Spring gave way to summer, and for weeks I dutifully logged in hundreds of miles on my bicycle. Although bewilderingly repetitive in the short term, in the grand scheme of things it made perfect sense: On a multi-day ride, if I am riding fifty to a hundred miles per day, I needed to be adequately prepared to handle a myriad of temperatures, weather and road conditions. As RAGBRAI approached, my trepidation and anxiety steadily grew. *What if I don't have what it takes to finish the week? How will I handle the rolling and steep inclines and the brutal July heat in the middle of Iowa? Will I make a fool of myself because I cannot keep up with the other riders?*

At last, the final week in July arrived, and I had completed a successful season of training. All of the long hours under the warm sunshine had caused my arms and legs to become bronzed, but only from the middle upper arms and mid-thighs outward, a classic "biker's tan." After logging over one thousand miles in three to four months with increasing speed and improving endurance, I felt ready. As I rode my team bus west past the towns and farms of my native state along Interstate 80, central Iowa's concrete aorta, I nervously contemplated the fitness challenges and special memories which awaited me. Regardless of what would take place over the next week, I realized that I would be changed by the experience.

Early Sunday morning arrived, and after quickly taking down our tents and packing our duffels, our team set forth on our first ride of the week, a fifty-mile ride from Sioux City to Ida Grove. It was 5:45 a.m., and the cool dampness of the early morning was about to be disrupted by a rapidly ascending sun, with a corresponding quick increase in temperature. We got off to an early start, knowing that the first day of bicycling would be quite hilly with temperatures into the 90's later in the afternoon.

As we rode out of the gentle, pastoral Missouri River Valley, and traversed the scenic and steep grassy khaki-colored Loess Hills to reach the western Iowa plateau, I rapidly felt my confidence increasing. I conquered every challenge that RAGBRAI threw at me that day, surmounting each daunting hill with astonishing ease, passing multiple riders on the upward climbs. All of the weeks of hard work and sacrifice spent on Wisconsin's rolling terrain were poised to pay big dividends. On a drought-stricken, prickly tan stretch of grass I pitched my tent in the scorching sun that afternoon. As I lazily drifted off to sleep under a speckled dazzling canopy of abundant stars that night, I reflected on a wonderful special first day's worth of memories. I marveled that I didn't feel any pains, headache or extreme fatigue. I became optimistic that RAGBRAI would be a triumphant, valedictory ride.

Straddling my sparkling jet-black Trek road bike the next morning, I reviewed the day's route on a laminated index card. Seventy miles, due south from Ida Grove to Audubon. Only four towns to pass through and navigate, the amount of hills and climb was slightly easier than yesterday's journey, and it was spread out over twenty more miles. It appeared to be very feasible and did not represent a formidable obstacle on paper.

As the day wore on, however, a couple of worrisome trends emerged. First, a gentle breeze appeared stealth-like early in the morning, steadily increased, and by afternoon reached 25 mph out of the due south. It proved to be a devastating, fierce headwind, which on a oppressive July day felt like it was emanating from an immense blast furnace. Polite conversations often shared between the riders began to dwindle and faded into oblivion as in despair we huddled over the handlebars and attempted to reduce our anatomical profile against the stiff breezes. Temperatures escalated into the low 90-degree range, and to compound misfortune, the humidity rapidly followed suit. The air became oppressively hot and heavy, and the dreaded "4-H" tetrad of heat, headwind, hills and humidity began to take their toll. I had trained for multiple contingencies on RAGBRAI, but only for one calamity at a time. Unfortunately, we were facing a serious quadruple challenge in the context of an unfamiliar location and situation.

Even the downhills were not very helpful. Cyclists desire rolling hills or a slope profile with a quick decline and incline, a so-called V-shaped valley. On those types of hills, the cyclist can develop enough momentum to reach about halfway up the successive peak, saving some energy. This was not to be on this Black Monday. The valleys in western Iowa tended to be more box-like, or U-shaped, obliterating any downward momentum on the prolonged flat river bottom. The headwind sabotaged what little kinetic energy remained on our two-wheeled machines. It had become an afternoon of severe struggle and a battle of which indomitable wills would survive the ultimate ordeal.

We were still about ten miles away from our final destination in Audubon. I had gone through twelve bottles of water and Gatorade, and felt my mental and physical endurance inevitably slipping away, like steam abruptly vanishing into a vast expanse of air. As I glumly pedaled in a disconcerting silence, I engendered a negative thought which would have been unthinkable just twenty-four hours ago.

I don't think that I can do this for much longer . . .

In desperation, I frantically scoped around the landscape, looking past orange rusted old windmills and brown weathered fences, hoping to find some inspiration to break this serious mental breakdown. And just like that, I found my focal point . . . in a cornfield. My RAGBRAI dream paralleled the story of an Iowa corn plant. It began small like a seed buried in the topsoil, in the darkness, uncertain and apprehensive. As I broke down my body and built it back up to ideal conditioning, the corn seed was shattered to sprout small shoots of hopefulness. Nurturing spring rains and summer sunshine ensured that the cornstalks

177

were vibrant and strong; and regular training rides were essential for me to develop strength and mental toughness. Adverse moments of personal discouragement and burnout, like severe thunderstorms and drought, frequented the journey, but were only transient. Finally, at the end of the process and growing season was the glorious autumnal harvest of accomplishment— the transformed auburn rows of maize, heavily laden with their bountiful yield of ears of corn. A rich reward for my tremendous personal investment and an athletic job well done awaited me. Contemplating that powerful motif, I was determined not to let my RAGBRAI dream plant wither and die that day and persevered through those last ten brutal miles.

Demoralized, we limped into camp at about 2:30 p.m. Despite being only early afternoon, it had been a long, difficult trek. I expected us to be among the last group of riders into camp upon completion of that horrible day. Instead, at our team's campsite we were greeted by a huge pile of duffel bags: As opposed to being amongst the stragglers, we were actually part of the early bird group.

After cleaning up and pitching our tents, we went to the local Methodist church for an early spaghetti dinner. As I absently shifted the pasta, sauce and meatballs on my burgeoning plate, I was discouraged and fearful—*Only my second day on RAGBRAI ever, and I barely finished out the day?* How was I ever going to get through an entire five-hundred-mile week of cycling? Despite thousands of fellow riders, we were in one of the most sparsely populated regions of Iowa.

I contemplated my options: continuation versus abandonment, and came to the identical conclusion that innumerable other exhausted cyclists reached in their tents that night—the show would go on. Day three would begin tomorrow morning, and it would commence and proceed whether I remained involved or withdrew back home to Wisconsin. The obvious solution was to ride again tomorrow and take on that day's challenges as they arose. On the road early the following morning, I felt reassured as I learned from numerous other veteran riders that yesterday's "Death March to Audubon" would go down in the annals of RAGBRAI history as one of the most difficult riding days on record.

The final day of the ride was a gentle, rolling fifty-mile ride from Iowa City to the Mississippi River town of Muscatine. Early that morning I pedaled up the hill past the University of Iowa, including the historic Old Capitol building with its glittering golden dome, my old stomping grounds. I recalled how over eight years at the university I grew and changed as a person, and similarly, my first RAGBRAI ride had done the same for me.

As I approached the final miles of my weeklong journey, I caught a mirrored image of my appearance in a storefront window. At that moment I realized that my long quest was almost completed, and everything seemed so clear. It was in that self-portrait within that glass reflection that I found it: *The virtual talisman of manhood hanging from my tanned and leathered form, which I dreamed about in my dark days!* My physical condition was fit and strong, bolstered by an intense week of riding under multiple stressful circumstances, a dream birthed from way back in the spring on the chilly, windswept moraine hills of Wisconsin. When I ceremoniously dipped my front tire in the Mississippi River, ending the weeklong journey, I was exhilarated by my accomplishment. Whenever I struggle with exhaustion and discouragement in the course of daily living, I take personal inspiration in my ability to steel myself to overcome these challenges like that hilly, oppressively warm July bicycle ride in western Iowa.

Whether presenting as part of an unusual medical condition, forming a fond patient memory, or marking a hallmark transition in personal fitness, like a fine treasured antique, my bronze memories hold a special place in my soul. Its deep, sepia metallic hues serve as a reminder to be aware of subtle yet important attributes of my patients and my physical being, and truly appreciate the rich beauty in unexpected people and places in the world.

CHAPTER 13

DARKNESS

M y Grandma Helen was resilient and strong, somewhat from inner desire, partially out of pure necessity. She grew up on a small Iowa farm, working to help pay her way through Central College to receive her education degree and teaching certificate. As a country schoolteacher in the cold, heartless teeth of the Great Depression, she received an annual salary of $360 in 1933. She lovingly toiled in the rural school system around our county, not only teaching, but also serving as schoolhouse custodian and caretaker.

Being happily married and having the gift of a job were an insufficient refuge from further struggles. Her husband developed a brain tumor, a terrible and challenging diagnosis at any age, but especially in the late 1940s. The malignancy was inoperable, progressed and maliciously took my Grandpa Herman in the prime of his life at the age of thirty-seven. Having lost the love of her life, Helen faced an existence as a single mother, with the daunting prospect of raising her three-year old daughter alone.

Fortunately, her parents stepped in, and she moved with them off the farm and into town for a fresh start. In the mid-twentieth century, single motherhood was not commonplace and not often perceived as a socially acceptable way of life. Through the multifaceted stressors of grief, financial uncertainty and parenting, my grandmother persevered and carved out a life for her family.

After moving into a small modest home in my hometown of Oskaloosa, she began teaching fourth grade at Jefferson Elementary School, a position that she would hold for the remainder of her thirty-eight-year teaching career. Upon her retirement, she had inspired and intellectually stimulated hundreds of elementary school children. Many of her former students have proclaimed to me that Mrs. Helen Douwstra was by far their favorite teacher. It was incredibly flattering and humbling to realize that someone close to me had such an intimate and profound impact upon other childrens' educations.

What most people did not know was that Helen silently suffered from multiple, intermittent bouts of depression. Perhaps because of the social stigma associated with mental illness in that era, her perceived need to keep moving on with life, or a desire to be at her best for her students, my grandma was not open about the internal turmoil which confronted her. She often said that she "wept for months" after my grandfather passed away. Grandma's relatives frequently spoke in hushed tones about Helen's depression and need to take her "nerve medicine."

None of this made sense to me. How could my grandma be depressed? She took me for ice cream and to stop by the railroad tracks to watch the diesel trains thunder through town. We created outlandish craft projects and spent hours playing virtually every board game imaginable. Everyone loved her enthusiasm for living and teaching, and the projected joy of her personality, even if somewhat superficial, was infectious. Melancholy and depressed people, in my middle school mind-set, were weird; they cried all of the time, could not function in daily life, and often needed to be institutionalized. An amazing woman such as my grandmother certainly did not fall under the category of someone struggling with a mental illness.

In retrospect there were multiple subtle signs that my grandma suffered from a chronic mood disorder. She occasionally without warning would appear withdrawn, became melodramatic at times, and would frequently get angry and tearful at seemingly inconsequential situations. Because of my grandma's pride and private nature regarding her psychiatric issues, she was undermedicated and occasionally not on any pharmacological treatment at all for anxiety or depression. In those days, the drugs available for treatment were limited, of inconsistent efficacy and had frequently had side effects. The more modern medications, including the serotonin selective reuptake inhibitors (SSRIs), were one to two decades away. She never received counseling for these troubling issues on an ongoing basis.

Her ability to continue working at a high level, while caring for her family and successfully maintaining a household without these external supports, was a testament to her indomitable personality. Her ongoing educational legacy to me as a practicing physician was to be vigilant for subtle signs of mood disorders, treating them promptly with medication and psychotherapy, hopefully avoiding Grandma's lonely journey.

In late April of 1973, I sat glumly in my grandma's front room staring out the window. We had planned a nice picnic in the park, including playing on the swings and slides. However, Mother Nature refused to cooperate, and a typical spring downpour derailed our plans. Rain torrentially drilled downward in intense, shimmering sheets, obliterating all hope of doing anything enjoyable outside. Rivulets of raindrops danced and cascaded down the windows, mocking my melancholia. As a five-year-old boy, my grandmother and I played together for hours and created multiple crazy, make-believe adventures. Usually those types of activities were enough to assuage my disappointment about being cooped up inside.

Around noon, my mom came over and we had chicken noodle soup and grilled cheese sandwiches. By the mid-afternoon, it was time to head for home. However, in order to reach our car, we were going to have to brave the merciless deluge outside. Mom had just had her hair done and got a plastic baggie to put over her head. Seeing that she had something to keep her head dry, I wanted a bag also—she procured one and placed it gingerly onto my thick sable hair. I gave Grandma a kiss goodbye and we raced out the door.

As we sprinted the relatively short distance toward our car, a sudden fierce updraft emanating from the storm buffeted us, and tore the frail plastic bag from my hands and off my head. It sailed momentarily upward and across the busy highway in front of the house, before unceremoniously crumpling down onto the saturated pavement. The gossamer bag now was lifeless on the four-lane highway, saturated by the downpour and crushed by the repetitive unknowing passing vehicles. By this time, we had made it into the vehicle, and my mom, seeing that I had lost my head covering, with a sweet gesture placed hers onto my head.

This was the last straw, it was all too much. The picnic in the park, having fun at the playground, swinging with all my power to touch the blue sky with my feet . . . it had all been swept away in the cruel rainy-day torrent. When I tried to protect myself from the elements, the malevolent storm took that away too. I felt a disconcerting tickle in my nose, a clear upwelling in my eyes, and a cascading downpour of emotions. The tears came fast and furiously, followed by my cries of frustration and utter heartbreak.

"This is so unfair! We couldn't do anything today because of the rain! I hate the rain! I hope it never rains again! If it never rains again, we could have fun outside, and I'd be happy and never sad!"

My mom didn't respond to this diatribe immediately, and clearly she was not mutually experiencing my anger and sadness. Rather, she quietly turned to face me, as I sat wet and dripping under my makeshift plastic hood. Her round, almond dark-brown eyes kindly fixated on me. A calming sense of contentment projected from her, and her face appeared to be bright, incongruous, almost smiling against the dark-gray backdrop of the gloomy tempest raging outside our vehicle's windows. She spoke to me in a soft, genuine voice in a manner that I had never heard from her.

"Bruce . . . with no rain there'd be no flowers in our garden, no food for us to eat, no drinking water, and no swimming pools. So no matter how rainy the day is, remember rain is also important and a sunny day will be here tomorrow, OK?"

Even at the age of five, I marveled at the power and sensibility of my mother's thoughts in that moment. I looked up at her humbly and with a slight lessening of my depressed emotions. The tears stopped, and through my synthetic waterlogged chapeau, I simply stated, "OK Mommy, tomorrow will be better." My mom smiled comfortingly, started the car, and we headed for home. As a grown man, I fondly recall the rainy-day childhood lesson from my mother, and strive for sunny optimism during phases of clouded tribulation.

It was 6:00 a.m., and my pager, with its shrill warble, rousted me from my short reverie of sleep in my spartan, utilitarian call room at Waukesha Memorial Hospital. As a second-year resident, my 24-hour shift of OB call was one hour from being complete, and I would be free to go home for some rest. The Labor and Delivery main desk was looking for me. I threw on my white lab coat over my green scrubs and walked the short distance to the birthing center main station. When I had headed to my cot at around 4:00 a.m., the unit was almost empty, the whiteboard of record devoid of any black marker scripting.

Upon my arrival on the unit, I was not greeted by the typical smiles or "Good morning" from the staff. The unit clerk looked at me with an air of significant concern and worry creasing her face. She regarded me sternly, completely out of character for her normal demeanor, and tersely stated, "Room 22 . . . now!"

The entire atmosphere of the ward seemed to be permeated with a sense of negative energy and impending doom. I intangibly grasped it, and made my way down the hallway to the only expectant mother on the floor. As I entered Room 22, there were four nurses gathered around a sweet young couple. The anticipatory excitement and happy moods normally indigenous to these pre-delivery situations had evaporated. Throughout the room an air of worry and concern was palpable, almost suffocating in fear that something wasn't right with this mom and baby.

I completed a brief nonverbal survey of the room, collected my thoughts, and delicately approached this sensitive situation. "Hi, I'm Dr. Rowe, the resident on call for tonight. What's your name, ma'am?"

"Connie McMillan," replied the expectant mother, with a prominent fearful tone in her voice.

"What's going on right now?" I queried the care team.

Jackie, a seasoned lead L&D nurse, spoke first. "Dr. Rowe, we're having a hard time getting heart tones with the fetal heart monitor, and when we do, the rate is quite slow, about 70 beats per minute." This pulse rate *was* significantly lower than normal. Normal healthy, reassuring fetal heart rates range typically around 120–150 beats per minute.

Immediately, I performed a discrete, bedside cervical check examination. She was 4 cm dilated, but more ominously a copious amount of meconium exuded from the vaginal canal. Meconium is the medical term for newborn baby poop; often it is a signal that a baby is experiencing potential significant intrauterine distress.

"Who's the overnight on-call OB attending physician?" I asked.

"Dr. Finley is on tonight," came the nursing reply.

"Did you guys page her yet? She needs to get in here now!" I found myself struggling to maintain composure.

"Yes, already done. She'll be here urgently in about ten minutes."

OK, so I have ten minutes to get this figured out before she gets here. "Alright, I need a fetal scalp electrode, and the bedside ultrasound machine here immediately!"

Jackie handed me the electrode. It was a long length of wire with a small spring sensor electrode on the end, which is harmless to the baby. It allowed me to more accurately assess the baby's true pulse status. I quickly and gently corkscrewed the electrode onto the baby's scalp, and changed the setting on the fetal heart monitor. Almost immediately, the beeping sounds of the heart rate called out to me, and I could tell even without checking the digital readout the heart rate remained still too slow, at around 70–75 beats per minute. At that point the ultrasound machine arrived at the bedside. I squirted a dollop of gel onto Mrs. McMillan's protuberant belly and ran the sensing transducer across it. I glanced at the images on the screen, and was struck at the activity of the baby's heart—it looked sluggish and devoid of the happy, jumping, hyperdynamic appearance that I was used to seeing on fetal ultrasound studies.

I was faced with a dilemma—this baby was in serious trouble. Do I call a crash C-section and take her back to the OR to perform the procedure myself, or do I wait a few more minutes for Dr. Finley and do this together? Despite first assisting on dozens of C-sections, I had never performed one myself, and doing one under incredibly stressful, emergent conditions didn't seem like a good starting point in my training. Furthermore, I reflected on my Hippocratic Oath and the key phrase in the entire passage—*primum non nocere*—"above all else, do no harm." I made the weighty calculation that I would cause more harm from my inexperience and lack of technical proficiency as opposed to benefiting mom and baby. Jackie was standing right beside me, keenly aware of the tenuous condition of this baby. The degree of worry and outright panic of everyone, including myself, was becoming almost unbearable.

"Please call the Section Team together now—we may need to do this quickly once Dr. Finley gets here."

Five minutes later, with efficient timing, Dr. Finley arrived in the room. I felt a slight sense of relief that she was here, but interestingly I was not comforted as much as I would have expected. I gave her a thirty-second synopsis of the situation, and after introducing herself to the patient and husband, she completed a cervical check—it was congruent with my assessment. By now, the fetal heart rate monitor was erratic in terms of picking up the baby's heart rate, a common finding with external sensors; but with a much more accurate internal fetal scalp electrode in place, another worrisome sign.

Dr. Finley repeated the bedside ultrasound examination, and at this juncture the absolute worst scenario had taken place. The heart was plainly visible, at a standstill, nonbeating, the four-chambered powerhouse devoid of all life. I gazed at the screen half desperate, praying for even a tiny bit of movement and contraction, and half angry at the desolate black egg-shaped oval that only a few minutes ago beat for the last time in an all-too-short lifespan. It's over . . . *Shit! Fuck!* Dr. Finley's eyes and poker face lost their battle of impartial clinical bearing and conveyed a deepening sadness. She attempted to compose herself, then gently grasped Mrs. McMillan's hand and spoke the words that no expectant mother should ever hear:

"I'm so sorry Mrs. McMillan, but I'm afraid your baby has died."

It was a seminal moment that I hope to never witness again in my medical career. The normal markers and reassuring reference frames of hope and love seemed to dramatically retreat and fall. A realization of the worst nightmare became apparent, and the penumbra of grief and loss cast its shadow over the labor and delivery suite. This was supposed to be a place of new beginnings and dreams, lifelong beautiful memories being created. I felt the cold, heartless reach of death enter the room and brutally envelop everyone within its grasp, but especially the McMillans. The father, shocked and bewildered, spoke first. "How could this have happened?" he cried, not asking anyone specifically in his surroundings. "We followed all of the recommendations, there were no problems with the pregnancy!"

"Oh my God! Our daughter's gone!" Mrs. McMillan cried through copious tears. "We have clothes, toys, a pink bedroom all set our for her! What are we going to do? What do we tell our parents?" She epitomized all of the despair and sadness encircling the family and the caregiver team. The parents had broached an infinite abyss of grief that would in some ways never be reconciled. As doctors, nurses and support staff, we felt a profound sense that we had failed this family and deprived them of a newborn treasure. Her name was to be Madison; now her impacts in the world would be on a death certificate, a tombstone, and an indelible branding of emotional pain on all of the unfortunate participants.

The tragedy played itself over the remainder of the day. Mrs. McMillan had the final indignity of needing to labor and deliver her lifeless child, physical pain being traded not for a joyous birth but rather for additional empty unfulfilled promises. Dr. Finley and I spoke with Madison's grandparents, whose shock and bereavement will be forever etched in my medical psyche. The lead nurse Jackie later confided in me that she had also lost a baby of her own at term, rekindling some deeply intimate and tragic memories.

For several weeks I felt a terrifying perception of being swallowed up by a tremendous sense of guilt and sadness. I possessed a persistent and unsettling sense that I should have done more to save Madison and help her mother. Madison's autopsy showed that she died of overwhelming sepsis, related to an infection from *Escherichia coli*. The attending neonatologist on call that fateful day kindly took me aside and told me that even if I had performed the Cesarean section on Mrs. McMillan immediately, most likely Madison still would have died of her severe infection within a few hours.

It was cold comfort for me. For weeks my overnight sleep was disrupted; I lay in bed at 3:00 a.m., looking up at the dark, lifeless ceiling, attempting a cosmic connection. *I'm sorry Madison, I did everything I could to help you and your mother (or did I?).* I visualized Madison's first steps, softball games, prom dates, true love, children of her own . . . none of those joyous prospects would ever come true for her. *Should I have done more? Or because of my technical inexperience, did the "do no harm" rule apply? Was it all my fault?* How would her family move forward? Would they be able to recover and emotionally invest in the effort to conceive, carry and deliver another child?

About fifteen months later, I was walking through labor and delivery to see a newborn baby when Jackie excitedly motioned over to me. "Dr. Rowe, go over to Room 15! The McMillans are back! They had a beautiful baby girl! Everything went perfectly—I'm so happy for them!" Her voice was the perfect blend of joy and thanksgiving. Tentatively, I went to the McMillan's room, knocked softly and politely walked in and offered my congratulations. I reminded them of our connection from that catastrophic winter early morning, and expressed my gratitude that this pregnancy went well. They were appreciative of my visit, but understandably guarded about reliving a difficult chapter in their lives on such a joyous day. Their newborn daughter was pink, beautiful and healthy; her name was Megan. Their relief and happiness was a spectacular counterpoint to the darkness which shrouded their previous trip to the labor and delivery unit.

I often remember that last encounter with fondness and remind myself that even in the darkest hours, a glorious beacon of hope and happiness awaits around the bend for everyone.

When my daily existence becomes incredibly challenging, with escalating feelings of depression and a creeping stealthy sense of hopelessness, the creature that I call The Monster arrives to cause me strife. I can picture his horrific image and wielding terrible power within the dark corners of my consciousness. He is hulking, dark, chiseled, large in form with an unknowable visage. Around him exudes a dark and foreboding miasma of doom and despair. If I grant him access to my deep emotions, his reach and impact reign supreme. His inherent and frighteningly accurate understanding of my fears and vulnerabilities appears to be overwhelming.

At 4:00 a.m., he awakens me to let me know that the day will be long and difficult, with plenty of existential threats to my well-being and confidence. He emphatically conveys to me negative thoughts of fleeting happiness, undeserved success, and the impossibility of finding contentment. The Monster knows my darkest misgivings, cultivates a sense of inferiority and sadistically enraptures my pessimism. Riding upon a steed of disenchantment, he brandishes a sword of self-pity and internal criticism, cloaked in an armor of depression and protected by a shield of impenetrable gloom. On the worst days of my hopelessness, he gallops toward me thunderously down the dark valley, eyes gleaming, delighting in my suffering, sword raised, shield forward, horse's nostrils flaring, menacing and prepared to strike. I recall my Grandma Helen's struggles with depression and I become discouraged. How can I get past my genetic predisposition toward unhappiness and overcome this battle with melancholy under seemingly unsurmountable odds?

Over the years, through my intermittent yet tumultuous battle with depression, I have figured out the inherent weaknesses within The Monster and how to confront and defeat the beast. Remarkably, I began to learn the obvious truth: The Monster was my own unfortunate creation through the negative energies of my mind and an impermanent sense of low self-worth. I ultimately discovered my power and capability to confront the pessimistic entity, destroy it and banish it to the dark dimensions of irrational thoughts and implausible nightmares. By focusing on my life's positives—loving family, good health and a great job—I put on the mantle of happiness and optimism and began to enjoin the battle for my collective internal peace. I defeated the negative energies in my emotional life by deploying the opposite positive weapons in the fight: overcoming darkness with light, fear with hopefulness, anxiety with optimism, self-pity with inward compassion. These were not easy objectives to achieve; it required a tremendous amount of personal self-reflection, counseling, and even antidepressant medication to bring myself back into emotional balance and peace.

In late summer of 2017, my friends and I embarked on a unique adventure to Hopkinsville, Kentucky, to witness the first solar eclipse visible from the U.S. Mainland in nearly forty years. With building anticipation, we camped out overnight on the grounds of a whiskey distillery, surrounded by fellow eclipse enthusiasts and the fertile aromatic tobacco fields.

The following day fulfilled the scientific astronomical prophecy. Over a couple of hours, the dark new moon progressively ate away at the visible surface of the sun until the brilliant sphere was completely occulted, with only the residual brilliant crown of fire being visible around a stark disk of pure blackness. For two and a half minutes the entire bluegrass countryside was bathed in a surreal glow of twilight, ultimately interrupted by a sudden intense burst of light from one solar corner as the moon's umbra began its catlike retreat. The level of brightness rapidly returned to normal levels, and within a few hours it felt like nothing unusual had occurred that day.

I took inspiration from the eclipse as my own life experience—bright moments temporarily interrupted by periods of uncertain, frightening darkness, returning to the light of joy and normality once again. It is important to live life with the confidence that even in one's darkest days, hopeful sunshine is ready to burst forth over the horizon.

CHAPTER 14

YELLOW

Culturally, the color yellow carries multiple connotations of excellence and shortcomings in society. The world-famous Tour de France bike race lead rider wears a bright yellow-colored jersey called the *maillot jaune.* Hopeful military families look to trees and lampposts festooned with lemon-colored ribbons for optimism for a soldier's safe homecoming. However, yellow can also convey an environment of a precautionary nature, such as in construction zones and traffic signals. Shades of maize may represent some of the negative elements in people and culture. Yellow journalism symbolizes grossly biased and inaccurate reporting in media outlets. When someone is branded as "yellow-bellied," it strikes at the heart of their character and paints them as a person lacking in fortitude and courage.

Jaundice is a medical term which is used to describe a generalized yellowing appearance of the skin. It is related to an abnormal accumulation of a bile pigment called bilirubin in the serum and tissues. This malady can occur at all phases of life, and the causes range from a benign variation of normal to imminently life-threatening. Given its external, widespread and definitive deviation from normal physical exam findings, it is a straightforward condition to identify. The golden, often jarringly bright discoloration is abrupt and results in a panicked phone call to the clinic with a subsequent urgent follow-up appointment.

Our firstborn daughter Allison was born on September 8th, a sunny and cool early fall day in southeastern Wisconsin. The pregnancy process had been completely uneventful. In contrast, the delivery and postpartum had been marked by some anxious moments—an urgent vacuum-assisted delivery to fend off an emergent C-section due to a dropping fetal heart rate. A rising bilirubin level then developed, related to breastfeeding, along with my daughter's blood type A-positive being incompatible with her mother's O-negative configuration. Inevitably, she developed a prominent yellow hue on day two of life, and her bilirubin rapidly increased to around 15mg/dL, with normal level being around 1.5 mg/dL.

Her pediatrician astutely recognized the issue and placed her in a blanket of special lights, and supplemented her breast milk with a daily bottle of formula. She had a condition known as physiologic or breast milk jaundice, a common, self-limited condition of newborns. Thankfully, her levels steadily declined back to a normal range within about seven to ten days. Much to my relief, her ruddy peach color returned, and she had no further issues with high bilirubin levels, without any alternative bizarre metabolic medical malady. In retrospect, the resolution was sudden, like a traffic light transitioning from yellow to red while rushing by in an automobile.

I was volunteering in the free medical clinic at our hospital in Ozaukee County when our new patient Anthony came in for an evaluation. He was about fifty years old, and based on initial appearances clearly was in trouble. He was moderately confused, poorly groomed and had a overly protuberant belly which was incongruent with his moderately atrophied limbs. What got everyone excited that night, however, was his color: He appeared to radiate a nearly neon banana glow which, rather than sunshiny optimism, instead portended a serious medical condition.

During my brief and occasionally incoherent interview with Anthony, he indicated that he drank about one and one-half bottles of vodka per day. Alcoholic patients are exceedingly skilled at deception and minimizing their true intake, so most likely he was drinking two to three times that amount. He had lost his job two years ago as a machine press operator, divorced one year ago, and only saw his teenaged son a couple of times per month. As a result, his personal life was in free fall with no signs of a redemption or recovery, and with an equally dramatic physical decline. I was startled on his examination to see the brilliantly yellowed whites of the eyes, and felt his firm, nodular liver edge extending down 4 cm below the end of the rib cage. His distended belly sloshed and echoed with the sounds of liters of fluid which had escaped his blood vessels and settled into the cavity of his abdomen, a medical condition called ascites. After much cajoling and coaxing, Anthony reluctantly agreed to be admitted to the hospital for further evaluation.

Upon admission, the dreadful tale of chronic alcohol abuse and self-neglect began to unravel and negatively impact Anthony.

A CT scan showed a large amount of fluid in the abdomen, a cirrhotic liver, dilated veins in the spleen and near the esophagus which could rupture and bleed at any time. I called my dear friend Dr. Ellerbee for a GI consult, who saw him immediately that evening. He was started on diuretic pills to reduce the fluid retention, and we closely monitored all of his electrolytes and liver function tests. An anti-anxiety medication called lorazepam was employed to prevent a life-threatening alcohol withdrawal.

By the following morning not much had changed in Anthony's condition. His weight declined only slightly, and the apple-shaped belly greeted me once again. Later that morning, Dr. Ellerbee inserted a needle under local anesthetic into Anthony's abdomen and drained nearly five liters of amber-colored fluid out of the abdomen, a procedure called a paracentesis. This provided some relief for our struggling patient, but unfortunately it was only temporary.

Anthony's successive days were a whirlwind of progressive decline. His bilirubin level, now markedly elevated, barely budged despite all of our clinical interventions. Almost overnight, the wellspring of ascitic fluid returned to the abdominal cavity, once again replenishing the chamber with its harmful and compressive liquid. His only minor blessing was that he showed no signs or symptoms of severe alcohol withdrawal. Other lab studies told a discouraging tale: His albumin level, a sign of protein nutrition and liver health, was dangerously low at 1.7 gm/dL—in normal healthy adults, it should be around 3.5–5.0. The liver also makes factors to facilitate clotting, and Anthony's clotting tests were significantly elevated despite not being on any blood thinners. This indicated that his failing liver was incapable of protecting him from bleeding. Finally, in the most grave of his metabolic setbacks, his kidney tests were now showing signs of deterioration; thus, now two major organ systems were failing. This complication is referred to as hepatorenal syndrome, a condition with a significant mortality rate.

As Anthony progressively declined, I was overcome with a pervasive sense of sadness and tragedy. Life's disappointments and setbacks led to his hopeless, destructive alcoholism, culminating in horrific irreparable physical damage to his body. It all seemed so senseless and preventable. He was not a liver transplant candidate, and given his circumstances, he made a difficult decision to not employ any aggressive measures to maintain his survival. He irrevocably slipped ever downward toward the cold, bitter embrace of death. In Anthony's final hours, his teenaged son paid a final visit, emerging from the room shell-shocked and horrified, crushed by the crippling weight of his grief. I secretly wished that some of my untreated alcoholics and problem drinkers would have witnessed the horrible scene that transpired that day.

On a cold, damp Sunday April afternoon, my wife and I were planting sapling maple trees in our backyard. My wife loves doing yard work, regardless of the weather conditions, even on a day which felt like the very antithesis of spring. Midway through the process, she began to note some increasing middle abdominal pain and cramping, culminating in her sitting down on the back patio stoop. I was befuddled and mildly irritated at her uncharacteristic behavior—our three young daughters were not capable of helping me. Annoyed and tired after planting the remainder of the trees myself, I checked in with Laura.

"How are you doing, honey?" I inquired, struggling to remain empathetic and conceal my frustration.

"Not so great, I have a lot of cramping and pain all over my stomach, maybe it was something that I ate," Laura replied.

"Take some Tylenol or ibuprofen, try something bland for dinner, and hopefully things will clear up over the next few hours."

Laura meekly agreed, and after a meal of some chicken noodle soup and toast, prematurely went off to bed for the night. The overnight hours were uneventful, and I was hopeful that the situation was resolved. When dawn arrived, it was apparent that Laura was not improving. She looked haggard, like she was attempting to make an internal mental and physical bargain with a persistent, ongoing level of discomfort.

"How'd you sleep last night, Laura?" I asked, now genuinely interested and concerned.

She gave me a worried and uncomfortable glance. "Terrible— the pain woke me up multiple times, I didn't sleep well, and the pain shot through to my back. Isn't that weird?"

It wasn't really weird so much as it was worrisome. People normally shouldn't have pain waking them up at night, especially people like my wife, who had birthed three kids without an epidural. Furthermore, the radiation of pain to the back suggested possibly a more pressing, serious intra-abdominal pathology. Laura needed to see the doctor today to sort out this potentially serious medical problem. I make it a point not to treat my family for most medical issues.

Later that morning, Dr. Jack Stephenson and my wife came over to my office for a brief medical consultation. His eyes effectively projected both concern and a sense of reassurance. "Bruce, Laura has gallstone pancreatitis. Her lab tests showed very high amylase and lipase levels, and an abdominal ultrasound showed a 1.5 cm gallstone in the bile duct, blocking the passage of bile and pancreatic fluid into the intestines." Glancing at my wife, I witnessed her tiredness and a slight yellowish discoloration of the whites of her eyes, from bilirubin accumulating from the blocked bile duct.

"We need to take care of this problem today," Jack stated emphatically. Laura and I agreed without hesitation

Subsequently, Laura underwent a procedure to dislodge retained stones in the bile ducts, followed by removal of her gallbladder a day later. In rare cases, pancreatitis can engender irreversible organ damage and culminate in death. Fortunately, she had an excellent gastroenterologist and general surgeon, and made a full recovery. It was gratifying to see my colleagues engage in positive collaboration to provide a high-quality medical experience for my wife.

A patient who arrives in the office with significant painless jaundice is frequently a disheartening situation. This almost always indicates a malignancy within the gastrointestinal system—pancreatic, gallbladder or bile duct cancers, for example. These diseases are a murderer's row of devastating oncologic problems, aggressive in nature, spreading quickly, detected late, and devoid of good curative options.

Charles was in his late seventies when he came in for an urgent care visit in early June. He loved being outdoors, so it was atypical for him to be in the doctor's office on a warm summer day. As I watched him step onto the scale for his weight and vital signs check, my heart sank; his entire body was an unmistakable brilliant marigold hue. He had no fever and stable vital signs. The extent of his jaundice in the absence of any associated examination findings or pain was discouraging.

"Hi Charles . . . I see clearly why you are here today. When did you first notice the color change?"

"About one to two weeks ago. I've never had this before, do you know what this could be?" he asked, more with an air of innocence as opposed to fear.

"I'm unsure, Charles," I replied, struggling to maintain composure, but fearful of an impending serious medical issue. "Let's run some tests today, and we'll get a better sense of the situation."

Over the next few days, the tragic drama unfolded. Along with high bilirubin levels, imaging studies showed Charles to have a bile duct cancer that was quite extensive and had spread throughout the entire abdominal cavity. No surgery, chemotherapy or radiation was going to improve his condition. A few days later, we discussed his findings, giving him some time to process the gravity of a cancer diagnosis. After a few contemplative minutes, he finally spoke.

"Wow . . . not what I wanted to hear, but I guess we all have to die of something. I wish that it could be something else, but that's not my call, that's God's. I've a lot to take care of at home and with my family, but I'm going to make this time count. I've actually been blessed with a pretty long and awesome life, a lot longer than many other people. I know I'm going to cry a lot and have some dark times, but I appreciate your honesty and support."

After that moving soliloquy, there really wasn't much else for me to add. "Hang in there, buddy," I replied with a tinge of futile optimism and hopefulness, "we're here for you and to help you through this." Over the subsequent six to eight weeks, I bore witness to Charle's physical decline in rapid fashion, his transition into hospice care, culminating in his passing. I was struck by his quiet and powerful dignity coping with the cruel medical hand he had been dealt in the last phases of his life. I wondered whether I would respond with a similar level of inner strength and dramatic poise if I received a bad medical report. Inspiring lessons provided by Charles and similar patients have guided me through the dark times on my life journey.

In medicine, much like English language grammar rules, there are always exceptions to most medical presentations, including the world of painless jaundice. Terry was a forty-five-year-old man, a distant acquaintance who lived in my community. He didn't like seeing doctors, and usually came in once per year for his general physical examination. However, the unmistakable citrine coloration throughout his body had goaded even a stubborn person like himself to make an urgent clinic visit.

During his examination, I tried to reassure myself that even though he was jaundiced, we haven't seen any weight loss, and I couldn't identify any liver enlargement, abdominal fluid or swelling of the legs. He almost looked too good to be having an issue with jaundice, given that the rest of his exam was reassuring. Nervously, I began the laboratory and diagnostic workup, and many surprises quickly emerged. While his bilirubin was elevated like all jaundiced patients, his other liver tests were normal, and a CT scan of his abdomen and pelvis were negative for any signs of cancer. What startled me, however, was his significantly decreased red blood cell count: His hemoglobin level was 5.6 gm/dL, and normal for a man is 15–17gm/dL. Terry had severe hemolytic anemia, a condition where an antibody was destroying his red blood cells and releasing the bilirubin pigment encased inside the cells throughout the body.

In this situation, while the jaundice itself was not life-threatening, the severe anemia could present a serious problem. We admitted Terry to the hospital, and with blood transfusions and prednisone he achieved a full response and resolution over a period of several weeks. Given all of the potential ramifications of the presentation of painless jaundice, this outcome certainly represented a best-case scenario.

It was mid-October, and I took advantage of the brilliant sunshine and clear skies to embark on a hike in the city park near my home. The day was cool, crisp and low in humidity, the quintessential fall day. Nearly all of the oaks, maples and hickory trees were approaching peak color. Their autumnal pigment palette contrasted with the dark blue-green of Lake Michigan. As I made my way along the dirt trail to an expansive bluff overlooking a spectacular lakeshore scene, I was enveloped and captivated by the fantastic coloration variety of the trees. The scarlet, auburn and yellow leaves cascaded along the path and onto me, lodging in my hair, coat and sweater.

It was a bittersweet moment, bearing witness to nature's ultimate natural firework display. It was the tacit acknowledgment of life's impermanence and that the cold, barren and seemingly lifeless months of winter awaited in the wings for their opportunity. I breathed in the clean air and basked in the brisk easterly breeze emanating from the vast expanse of Lake Michigan set in front of me. A solitary golden white oak leaf dangling above me quietly detached and settled, dove-like, upon my shoulder.

I thought of Charles, Anthony, my daughter Allison, among others, and reflected on the duality of jaundice and other unique conditions in medicine, sometimes temporary and normal, other times deadly. Their stories, like old newspaper clippings, may fade and yellow, but their powerful tales carry me forward. Winter is fast approaching, but so is spring, and like the last leaf on a dramatically exfoliating tree, I feverishly cling to the hopefulness that even in times of gathering cold and increasing hours of darkness, a golden glory awaits for all of my patients, yellowed or otherwise, in another time and another place.

CHAPTER 15

BLINDSIDED

In the winter of '82, my dad and I drove down to the hospital in Ottumwa on a Saturday afternoon to visit my mom as she convalesced from hysterectomy surgery. A moderate amount of snow lined the shoulders and ditches, but the roads themselves were completely clear of snow and ice. A gentle northeasterly breeze blew through the barren corn and bean fields, with feathery tendrils of snow gently dancing across the roadway. The skies were completely overcast, but with high light-gray clouds, and no ominous weather indicators were present. We had a nice visit with my mom, and I was relieved at her improved condition. Dad and I grabbed a quick bite to eat in the cafeteria and then set off for the half-hour return trip back home.

As we left the northern outskirts of Ottumwa and entered the countryside, the weather abruptly worsened. Darkness was beginning to settle in, and we were blindsided by an unexpected snowstorm, with large, heavy menacing snowflakes. Visibility steadily deteriorated to zero, and the gray-black roadway was replaced with an unpredictable icy and snowy slush. Our windshield was pelted with an endless volley of densely packed sleet and snow. I watched with increasing trepidation as our speed progressively decreased until we were barely moving forward. Navigation through the whiteout conditions was rapidly approaching impossible levels. Alternatively our car attempted to break into a skid, followed by a slow grinding sound of the snowy shoulder trying to pull us into its grip. Our mutual conversation quickly dissipated into a tense silence. I turned to my dad and spoke in a voice that sounded too timid for a thirteen-year-old:

"Dad . . . I'm scared . . ."

I'll never forget his response. "Yeah . . . me too."

That comment caught me off guard. *What? This is my father we're talking about here. He is my hero, the bravest person that I know. How could he be frightened? Boy, we might be really screwed here.*

"Maybe we should just turn around, Dad."

"Nah, let's just keep goin' for now."

A few miles down the road, our decision was made for us. The blizzard conditions made US Highway 63 impassable, forcing us to stay in the small town of Fremont. We called on some nearby friends who graciously opened their home up to Dad and me. I was grateful that we were in a warm home, safe and sound from the harsh, life-threatening maelstrom outside rampaging through the open plains. It was sobering and reassuring to discover that my father had fears and frailty just like me.

Two days later we brought my mom home from the hospital on plowed bone-dry roads, over the identical arteries which had recently threatened our safety when covered with snow and ice. Similarly, in medicine, I do my best to remain on guard for unexpected events and unusual patients. It only requires a single adrenalin-churning, thought-provoking oddity to broadside my monotonous contentment, demanding my complete attention and problem-solving abilities. I try to project confidence and coolheaded thinking in these circumstances, which is not always easy to accomplish.

I first met Harold in the Intermediate Care Unit of Columbia Hospital in Milwaukee, an upscale, tightly knit and highly regarded hospital in Milwaukee's near North Shore region. Dressing down on the weekends at Columbia meant wearing a sport coat *without* a tie, a warm throwback to the days of traditional medicine as practiced in the mid-1900s. Harold had been admitted from the emergency department after having been in two car accidents in as many days, now having developed some increasing confusional episodes. Being my partner's patient, Harold was not overly familiar to me. Initial lab studies and a head CT down in the ED were negative. I entered his room and introduced myself.

"Hi, Dr. Rowe here, I am covering this weekend for Dr. Matthias."

"Harold Reynolds, nice to meet you, wish it wasn't in this godforsaken place . . ."

"Can you tell me what's been going on, Harold?"

"I really don't know. I've had two car accidents, both minor fender benders, one on Thursday, and then another on Friday. Both times the other cars T-boned me on the left front quarter panel. Luckily the second one hit in the exact same place on my car, so I won't need two repairs. I thought both cars ran a stop sign, but the other drivers said it was my fault. I've always been a really good driver."

"Have you been a little bit more confused lately?"

"My wife says that I haven't been myself for the last few days, but honestly I don't really know what to think."

"Any vision changes, speech problems, areas of weakness, numbness, tingling, headaches, shakiness or other neurologic things that seem odd to you?"

"I haven't really noticed anything. Do you think there's a problem with my brain, Doc?"

"I'm not sure yet, I need to review your tests and examine you first."

Before I began my physical exam, I reviewed all of Mr. Reynold's test results. They all were normal, including his blood count, metabolic studies, vitamin levels and CT scans. His presentation seemed to indicate a neurological issue, but of what nature exactly? I ran through an abbreviated list of potential diagnoses. *Atypical migraine? TIA or stroke? Cerebral hemorrhage? Brain tumor?* Hopefully the exam would shed some some light on this diagnostic conundrum. His basic physical examination was normal, just the neurological exam remained.

I take pride in my ability to complete a comprehensive, reliable neurological examination consistently in a brief five to seven minutes. First, I assess the level of alertness of the patient.

If they answer questions correctly in terms of time, place and person, then the assessment is *alert and oriented to those three issues*, i.e., A & O x 3 for short. Next is an examination of facial structures, motor strength and sensation, a series of tests which assess cranial nerve function. Sensory and motor exams checked Harold's ability to feel pinprick and light touch, as well as muscle strength. Using my small reflex hammer, I lightly tapped on his elbows, knees and ankles, checking for a lightning-quick opposite muscle jerk in response. I had him use that finger to touch my outstretched finger and move back and forth to check coordination. The base of the reflex hammer swept underneath his foot to look for the Babinski's sign. A normal test showed the toes clustering and pointing down, positive has the toes pointing up and fanning out as wide as possible.

Up to this point, most of the neurological tests were normal with the exception of two unusual findings. I performed a test of the visual fields on Harold by wiggling my fingers on different sides of his peripheral vision and asking him to identify the moving digits. Interestingly, he never saw any of my finger-wiggling on the left side of his field of vision. Furthermore, with testing of the strength of his various muscle groups, it took some coaxing to get him to utilize his left arm and leg as strongly as the right. This could be a symptom of something called left-sided neglect, where someone has had a neurological injury to the right side of the brain, significant enough that they can ignore nearly one entire side of the body.

I began to synthesize a possible hypothesis that a serious brain issue may be causing his unusual presentation of left-sided neglect, confusion and left regional visual field loss. Thinking back to my neuroanatomy lectures from medical school, I attempted to formulate a possible central nervous system lesion. Suddenly, the potential answer came to me—*a posterior stroke involving the right visual cortex region!* An injury to that area would explain the left side visual loss and possible left-side neglect issue. A few hours later, the brain MRI confirmed my suspicions—a stroke in exactly the region of the brain of which I had hypothesized. This would explain Mr. Reynold's two car accidents where he went through an intersection and was struck on the left hand side. *He never saw the other cars coming!* He made a modest recovery, spent some time in a rehab facility, and, unfortunately, I lost track of him.

This case was gratifying to me because the patient history, physical examination and diagnostic tests acted together in harmonious trinity to arrive at an appropriate diagnosis. Although my patient had been blindsided by two accidents, I worked hard to prevent myself from being similarly surprised by an alternate diagnosis.

Anna Colangelo was an eighty-year-old woman, a retired high school math teacher who had been in my practice for the last several years. A few years ago, she developed a severe abdominal infection and obstruction related to a severe flare of Crohn's disease, an inflammatory condition of the intestines which occasionally can be life-threatening. She required an emergent surgery to remove parts of her small and large intestine, and required an ileostomy be placed. An ileostomy opening is created by a surgeon to allow small intestinal fluids to drain out of the body into a bag on the front of the abdomen. The first night Anna was in the ICU, I feared that she might be headed on her way out of the this mortal world. However, she surprised me and the other doctors with her rapid recovery, and within five days she had stabilized enough to return back to her residence with some assisted home care services. I arranged for Anna to follow up with me in the office within the next few days.

Anna's initial follow-up appointment in our office was largely uneventful, save for some mild postoperative pain and moderate frustration with now having to empty and change an unsightly bag of intestinal fluid on her abdomen on a regular basis. I tried to emphasize to her the positive aspects of her current medical situation: The surgery has corrected a life-threatening infection and obstruction, her inflammatory bowel disease problem was now in remission, and her strength and energy were increasing daily. She seemed cheered and buoyed by these observations.

Approximately one month later, I entered Anna's exam room expecting to see continued clinical progress, increased healing and decreased pain and concerns. Instead, I was surprised to encounter a patient who was visibly struggling to breathe.

"Anna, what's goin' on?" I inquired with an equal measure of urgency and concern.

"I don't know . . . what's happening . . ." Anna replied tentatively with long pauses between phrases. "The last couple . . . of weeks I just . . . cannot seem to . . . catch my breath . . . ." Every word and phonation seemed to required a supreme effort, and I wasn't sure how long she could maintain this level of communication.

I began to run through my list of questions for dyspnea, the medical term for shortness of breath. Sometimes, the term is abbreviated SOB, which reflects my feelings exactly when I encounter many of these struggling patients. I gathered myself and asked, "Any chest pain, swelling of your ankles, problems laying flat in bed to breathe?" An elderly patient with sudden shortness of breath . . . *This seems like a classic diagnosis of heart failure to me.*

Anna seemed to choose her words carefully. "I don't know . . . I seem to be just . . . short of breath . . . all of the time."

"Have you been traveling recently, laying in bed more, not drinking fluids or moving less around the house?" *Perhaps pulmonary embolus, a blood clot in the lung could explain the sudden difficulty in respirations.*

"No, not really . . . but since I am so tired . . . and cannot breathe . . . it is hard to move around . . . very much anyway . . ."

I redirected my questions toward another potential diagnosis. "Any fevers or chills, cough, dark bloody sputum, sounds of rattling or wheezing?" *Maybe this is a complicated pneumonia, and IV antibiotics and fluids are what she needs.*

"Nope . . . haven't really noticed . . . any of those things," she responded wearily and with an increasing sense of worriedness and alarm. *What is going on here?* I did a brief but reliable physical exam on Anna, and other than a few crackle sounds in her lungs, not much stood out to me.

I decided that I had seen enough. Anna was transferred to the hospital for a direct admission to a medical bed for a further workup. An ultrasound on her heart, called an echocardiogram, showed normal cardiac function without evidence of heart failure.

A computerized tomography (CT) scan of the chest showed no blood clots in the lungs, and no evidence of pneumonia. Initially, the lab results appeared to be normal, and I was beginning to feel that I was no closer to my diagnosis. About thirty minutes later, I received a phone call from the laboratory.

"Dr. Rowe, this is the lab . . . I have a critical lab result to report."

"OK, shoot."

"Mrs. Colangelo's bicarbonate is critically low at 8 mEq/L." Normal bicarbonate level in 24–32 mEq/L.

"OK, thanks." I hung up the phone and tried to wrap my head around this new piece of peculiar clinical information. *Why would her bicarbonate level be so low? Is she acidotic? What is causing this?*

Anna was clearly losing large quantities of bicarbonate which was adversely altering her pH balance. The triggering factor continued to be elusive to me. After a period of contemplation, I arrived at the solution: Anna had an ileostomy tube, and her body's bicarbonate ions were draining out en masse through her intestinal opening. A follow-up test called an arterial blood gas confirmed the severity of her acidosis and explained her shortness of breath: When people develop a metabolic acidosis, or excessively elevated acid levels in their blood, they respond by increasing their rate of respirations to help compensate.

Now I had a diagnosis and a reasonably clear pathway toward a clinical solution. I contacted a nephrologist, a doctor who specializes in metabolic diseases. We started Anna on sodium bicarbonate tablets three times per day, and within thirty-six hours her bicarbonate levels, respiratory rate and breathing distress completely returned to normal. Patients who unexpectedly present with shortness of breath are an unsettling medical situation. Although very common, not all episodes of respiratory difficulty are related to a heart or lung problem; sometimes in medically unclear situations it often requires an openness to alternative diagnoses in order to overcome the initial shock of a sick patient, quickly resolving their health concerns.

A few years ago a particularly virulent influenza outbreak, H1N1 subtype, viciously attacked the upper Midwest throughout the early spring season. Many of my older, debilitated nursing home patients were adversely affected by this malicious infection. Any suspicious case required us to wear a gown and a mask. It was the Friday of Memorial Day weekend, and the outbreak was at its peak. I was getting suited up to see my next possible influenza patient.

Stacy Liu was a nice fifty-year-old Asian female who was doing reasonably well until a few days ago, when she developed fevers to 102.0 degrees, chills, body aches and pains. Many of these cases over the last few weeks had proven to be influenza, and I was prepared to proceed with a diagnosis and treatment protocol that we had executed all-too-frequently recently.

Almost immediately after I began speaking with Stacy, however, it seemed like this situation was altogether different. I was blindsided by her atypical presentation—she had the fevers, chills and body aches that were hallmarks of influenza, but she was devoid of any cough, runny and stuffy nose that we would normally see in the setting of flu. In addition, she had no diarrhea or pain with urination, which if positive could have also explained her symptoms. Furthermore, and perhaps most critically, Stacy looked *sick*. Often in medicine, especially in pediatrics, an initial assessment on how sick a patient *appears* can shed some light into what might be a patient's problem. Her initial physical examination failed to reveal any specific causes for her illness, but clearly something medically significant was underfoot.

In a sense of desperation having arrived at a diagnostic impasse, I asked one of the few questions that I had remaining in my quiver. "Any other symptoms that you have noticed recently?'

"Well, I called my gynecologist yesterday, because I have a yeast infection and a sore bottom. She called in some medication in for me, but I don't think it has kicked in yet."

"Stacy, I think that we should have a look at your bottom today."

"Really? Do we have to? I really don't want to show you my private areas."

"I know it's awkward for you," I replied gently, "but this could be an important clue in figuring out your problem."

Reluctantly, she conscientiously disrobed, and my assistant and I prepared to complete a pelvic examination. However, upon visualizing her outer pelvic area, it was clear that no further assessment was necessary. What I saw externally there caught me completely by surprise: There, vividly displayed, was a large diffuse area of redness, swelling and pain, consistent with a large perirectal abscess. Based on her initial presentation and my current biases toward influenza diagnoses at that time, I was shocked at the ultimate cause of her systemic illness.

This was not a case of influenza; she was going to need to be hospitalized immediately to receive IV antibiotics and have the abscess drained. Later that evening the on-call general surgeon successfully released the dangerous pocket of purulent debris. She required a couple days' stay in the hospital, and after a brief scare with an episode of sepsis made a full recovery. Focus and diligence prevailed, allowing us to arrive at the correct diagnosis when there were several opportunities to be thrown off track.

Maggie was a regular visitor to our emergency department at Presbyterian Hospital in Philadelphia. She was homeless and contending with the twin mental health issues of schizophrenia and bipolar affective disorder. Occasionally she would see us for significant clinical problems such as pneumonia and urinary tract infections. Other times, she just needed a warm meal, a place to sleep or shelter from a winter storm.

On an unseasonably warm April afternoon, Maggie made an unsurprising encore appearance. As a first-year intern, I had already worked with her once before for another ER visit. Today she came in for a fall with some left wrist pain, and her X-ray revealed a radial and ulnar fracture. She was going to need a splint applied prior to seeing the orthopedic doctor in the morning. I generated a flimsy worst-case scenario to the admitting hospital resident to justify Maggie's inpatient admission, then set to work placing her splint. Luckily, she was cooperative with me as I molded the fiberglass support into place.

"OK Maggie, I'm going to finish wrapping up this splint for you. We'll get you a sling for you to use, and then the ortho doctor will see you in the morning."

"Sure thing, Doc, thanks. Ah'm glad that ah'm here, it's a scary place out there. The government and the dark soldiers are all out to get me. They wanna erase my memories and make me obey."

"Oh Maggie, you're safe now, I really don't think tha—"

"You don't understan' Dr. Bruce, these people and organizations are really bad. They'll come for you, too, if you not careful. You're gonna need to protect yo' self."

"How're you going to protect yourself?" I curiously queried.

"Come here closer, I'll show you," she beckoned me mischievously.

Interested and wary, I engaged her request. She reached into her oversized, unbelievably weathered duffle and procured her weapon of choice. I was blinded momentarily by the seriousness of her actions and the bright reflection from the menacing serrations of what proved to be a nine-inch kitchen knife! "See here? Ah got this thing here for protectin' me."

I tried my best to conceal my sheer terror at the dangerous implement she brandished in front of me, despite a lack of direct threat. After I composed myself and confirmed that I was between her and the door, I subtly made my proposal.

"Hey Maggie, can I take that knife and put it away someplace safe until you get out of the hospital?" I inquired as innocently as possible.

"Oh sure, Doc, no problem, ah know ah'll be safe in here."

I gently took the knife and held it by the very top corner of the handle with my first and second fingers, like I was carrying a dirty diaper. Quickly I walked out to the nurses' station and made eye contact with my favorite nurse, Nancy. She was seasoned from many years of working crazy, stressful shifts in an inner-city ER. As I approached her holding the knife, even her jaded eyes widened dramatically, her mouth gaped open.

"Hey Nancy, can you take this knife away and put it someplace safe? Maggie brought this in and it's makin' me real nervous."

"Holy shit, Bruce! She didn't threaten you with that thing, did she?"

"Oh goodness no, she's having more delusions lately, and I think she kept it to feel safe."

"Uh . . . yeah, let's get this scary thing outta here." Nancy walked down the hall with the terrifying piece of cutlery. I never saw it again, and to my knowledge Maggie never asked for it back.

Caring for mentally ill patients is often fascinating, even to the point of being blindsided by patients' reactions to their all-consuming delusional thoughts. Being unpredictably broadsided by patient encounters and events can be simultaneously stimulating and terrifying. I have discovered that being adaptable and current in my medical knowledge has kept me composed and confident to confront turbulent medical situations.

CHAPTER 16

WEIRD

On nearly a daily basis, the peculiar aura of weirdness permeates the medical world. Patients often possess quirky or noncompliant behaviors. Physicians are attached to rituals in their schedules to the point of being obsessive-compulsive. Patients can present with unusual symptoms and tangential case histories, foiling a physician's best efforts to make an accurate diagnosis and deliver quality patient care. Weirdness can even take on the form of a bizarre or interesting case or person, something completely unanticipated, a rare or at least quirky diagnosis. These interactions never fail to grab my attention and keep life and the practice of medicine ever mysterious and occasionally entertaining.

In midwinter of my transitional internship in Philadelphia, I was hard at work in our inner-city emergency department one Friday evening. ED shifts are the ultimate crapshoot, a crazy tapestry quilt of quiet boredom, sheer terror and weird interactions. This particular shift had been a middle ground of busyness, enough to keep us on our toes without becoming overwhelming. I was finishing up some paperwork with the nurse when a tremendous commotion arose from the front entrance.

"Get him into Trauma 2 stat! I don't think he's breathing!"

"Where's Dr. Campanelli? Is Dr. Rowe back there?"

I sprung to my feet and ran into the trauma bay off to the right of the main entrance where they had wheeled the unfortunate patient. My lead physician Dr. Susan Campanelli and I hit the door simultaneously.

"What's goin' on guys?" she quickly asked the paramedics.

"We found him outside on the street corner, some passersby said that he looked confused, and then stopped breathing. No ID, no other info." They were vigorously bagging him with oxygen, but the patient still looked blue. He was hooked up to the monitor, and the patient had a pulse, albeit slow, and a very low oxygenation level of 65 percent—normal should be a solid A grade of 95 percent plus. As I frantically contemplated the nature of this emergency, Dr. Campanelli barked out a couple orders.

"Alright, we already have an IV started, let's bring the code cart over. I need Narcan 1 mg IV and Atropine 1 mg IV stat!"

My attending was acting on a hunch. Narcan is used to reverse opioid overdoses, which was a less common issue back then as it is unfortunately today. The atropine would stimulate his heart and increase his pulse rate. With stunning efficiency, the ED nurse accessed the IV and administered the two drugs. The next step was to sit back and wait for a few tense moments.

Our patient's response was dramatic and rapid. With lightning swiftness, our unknown patient sat bolt upright on the hospital bed.

"What the hell happened? What's goin' on?" he cried out.

I stepped in and tried to offer reassurance. "You stopped breathing, we treated you for a narcotic overdo—"

"That son-of-a-bitch set me up! He gave me some bad shit and took all of my money! I'm out $400! Where the hell is he? I'm gonna fix him good!" Abruptly he jumped off of the gurney, ran down the ED hallway, IV catheter still in his arm, right out the front entrance and back on the street once again.

I stood there transfixed, trying to digest the weird dramatic production which had just occurred. My emergency department brethren set aside their momentary disbelief and methodically cleaned up the room and moved on to the next case.

Dr. Campenelli politely sized me up as she walked out of the room. "Don't be so surprised, Bruce, this isn't as strange as you think. Remember, we work in an inner-city hospital, and we're all veterans of some pretty crazy stuff. Just watch and learn, OK?" She flashed an ironic smile and winked, patted me on the shoulder and briskly walked down the hall, unmoved by what took place. *This guy was dead on arrival and ran out of here five minutes later! No name, no thanks, no nothing.* It was an early in-training kickoff to a lifetime of medical oddity.

On a balmy summer day in the park, where my coworkers and I were having a cookout, two motorcyclists pulled up about a block away. However, about thirty seconds later one of the riders fell to the ground and began writhing and convulsing uncontrollably, in visible distress. I caught the disturbance in my peripheral vision with an accelerating level of concern. A couple of our nurses were already sprinting over the short stretch of parkland to the struggling motorcyclist. I urgently jogged toward the commotion, buying myself some time to consider potential diagnoses. A seizure disorder seemed most likely, given his behavior. *Severe headache? Brain bleed?* Some other source of pain or distress like a ruptured cerebral aneurysm seemed less likely. A few moments later I reached the calamity and began an assessment.

"Hi, I'm a doctor, name's Bruce," trying to project a veneer of calm through the miasma of panic. "What's his name?" I asked his riding buddy.

"His name's Phil," was the reply. "Apparently he's got something in his ear that really hurts."

"What's happenin', Phil?" I gently inquired.

"Holy shit! There's somethin' like a bug in my right ear! I think it flew in there when I was ridin' a few minutes ago. All I know is it hurts like absolute hell!" he screamed out and resumed thrashing on the ground.

A bug? Well, the mechanism of injury seemed plausible. Bikers strike insects of varying caliber all of the time. But Phil's reaction to the suddenly intruding insect seemed severe and disproportionate. Briefly, I contemplated my options. We had nothing in terms of medical equipment at our disposal. No otoscope to directly examine the ear, and no forceps to remove any potential foreign body from the external ear canal. I advised my nurse to call the EMS for assistance while I considered my next move. Neurologically he looked intact and conversant, so it did not appear to be a seizure or other central nervous system insult. He continued to focus on his affected ear, and noted no other areas of pain on his body. *Now what, Bruce?* I began to formulate a possible solution to the dilemma.

"Hey—you guys have any water bottles and a toolbox handy?" I asked the friend as Phil once again was struck with a paroxysm of pain, unmitigated thrashing of his limbs and grabbing at his right ear.

"Yes—I'll go get 'em . . . you guys gonna be able to help him?"

"We're sure gonna try," I countered cautiously.

I surveyed the equipment handed to me. A bike squeeze water bottle, perfect to direct a jet of water into the ear. The toolkit proved to be much less fertile ground for a helpful instrument— the only potentially useful implement was a simple #2 pencil. It would have to do for this predicament.

"Now Phil," I slowly enunciated with encouragement, "I need you to lay back down on your side with your left ear on the ground and your right ear pointing up to the sky. Can you do that for a couple of moments?"

"OK, I'll do my best." Phil's onslaught of severe pain seemed to be abating for a brief period. We were going to have to work fast.

I used the cycling bottle to steadily drip water into the ear canal, hoping to draw the malevolent critter to the surface. A few seconds later, my efforts were rewarded—a creepy, multi-legged bug, ironically an earwig, flashed briefly at the external ear opening before elusively diving back into the cool comfort of Phil's auditory canal. Doggedly, I continued to deliver water into the insect's sanctuary until it made an encore appearance. This time I was ready, and with the plain pencil in my right hand deftly swept the minuscule crawling creature completely out of the ear canal.

With the removal of the troubling impacted insect, the change in Phil's demeanor was stunning and dramatic. His pain had totally vanished, and now he quickly stood up and smiled with a obvious lightening of his discomfort levels.

"Thanks Doc, I appreciate that. It's all better now."

"You're welcome. No problem." I stood there stunned at the complete reversal in circumstances from just one to two minutes ago. *Wow . . . what on earth was that all about? That must have been one hell of a bug problem in that ear.* By the time the paramedics had arrived we had the embarrassing yet satisfying opportunity to send them away without any further intervention. I learned that when encountering unusual medical crises out in public, sometimes you have to improvise to achieve results.

Atypical medical presentations can also be serious, with less fortunate end results. Clifford came into the office as a new patient early in my career as a family physician. He noted some increasing left hip pain, but denied any history of trauma or surgery to the affected areas. My physical examination showed some generalized hip pain and slight decreased range of motion, otherwise negative. I ordered a set of X-rays, expecting to find the unmistakable loss of joint space and bone spurs associated with osteoarthritis.

The films ultimately revealed some arthritis, but not to the degree that I was expecting based on his symptoms. Furthermore, the pelvic bone region around the left hip area looked strange—an area of Swiss cheese appearance which definitely could explain his symptoms. As a result, I concluded that two main categories of diagnoses were possible—either metabolic problems disrupting normal bone turnover such as Paget's disease or, more ominously, metastatic disease from cancer. His subsequent bloodwork was negative for any bone metabolism issues, and the tumor markers for cancer were normal with one glaring exception: The prostate-specific antigen test, normally registering a level at around 1–4, was tremendously elevated at over 9,000! It was the highest PSA level that I had ever witnessed. Follow-up rectal exam showed a markedly enlarged prostate, nodular with branching tendrils of tissue which gives cancer its crab-like nomenclature. A biopsy confirmed a diagnosis of prostate cancer.

Because his malignancy was so advanced, Clifford was not a candidate for surgical removal of the prostate. His oncologist initiated hormonal drugs designed to prevent testosterone from progressing the prostate cancer. The astronomically elevated PSA level declined from 9,000 down to 50. A few months later, Clifford returned to me for a follow-up visit. I was pleasantly surprised at his ebullient mood and improved mobility.

"Hello Clifford," I began, "you look great today, how's it going?"

"Feelin' a fair amount better now. Dr. Klein has me on good meds to knock out the cancer. I can now walk without my hip hurtin' and spend some quality time with my grandkids. Thanks, Doc, for figurin' out my problem."

"You're welcome, Cliff. Hope you keep moving as well as you are right now."

"Sounds good, I'll see you around, but hopefully not too soon." With that, he arose and departed with a newfound level of confidence and stability. Watching from behind, I noticed that his gait was secure and free of limping. Clifford lived for an additional seven years. His case was a tremendous illustration that some joint pains in elderly patients can have weird causes and not necessarily be from osteoarthritis.

Brandon was an active ten-year-old boy who came into the office with his mother on a brutally hot and humid summer day. He had fallen onto a stone in the muddy waters of the nearby Milwaukee River, lacerating the front of his left knee. The cut was deep and widely gaping, but fortunately it was not actively bleeding. It needed to be sutured along with treating him for a contaminated water exposure. I irrigated the laceration with sterile saline, updated his tetanus booster, and stitched the wound closed. Next, I gave him a shot of antibiotics with ceftriaxone then sent him home with an oral antibiotic, Augmentin. As the visit concluded, I reassured myself that we had successfully prevented a secondary wound infection.

Two days later, my false vanity was shattered as Brandon unceremoniously returned to the office with the unmistakable signs and symptoms of a wound infection. He had a fever to 101.5 degrees, and the surgically repaired left knee laceration site was hot, swollen and tender. Brandon needed to be admitted to the hospital for IV antibiotics, with infectious disease and orthopedic consultation. Upon removal of the sutures, I was greeted by a moderate amount of watery, stinky yellow purulent fluid, which I sent for culture. After getting Brandon settled in the hospital I made the humbling ten-minute drive back home.

What am I missing? The wound was irrigated copiously, he was protected with broad-spectrum antibiotics. *Was there an unusual offending bacterial pathogen that I overlooked?* Augmentin should have covered most types of organisms found in freshwater ponds and rivers, but clearly it was insufficient. River water, clearly contaminated and dirty, has a vast panoply of potentially infectious bacteria, Gram-positive and Gram-negative bugs, anaerobic bacteria and even . . . *Aeromonas!* That last bacteria is atypical and would not have responded to his current antibiotics. With optimistic confidence, I instructed the nurse to add the antibiotic ciprofloxacin to his medication regimen. The following day, a positive *Aeromonas* wound culture confirmed my suspicions, and Brandon dramatically recovered within a couple of days. Brandon's clinical situation reminds me that when a patient is not improving, remain open to all potential diagnoses, even those of a seemingly weird and bizarre variety.

Margaret was a lovely thirty-five-year-old mother of two that I have cared for at least five years. We first met when she was pregnant with her oldest daughter Olivia, and I have maintained a special relationship with her family. She walked into the office with a sudden onset of significant facial spasm for the last twelve hours. As we exchanged our morning greetings, she was tight-lipped, brandishing an asymmetric and sheepish smiile.

"Hi Margaret, rough night last night, huh?"

"Yes, Dr. Rowe, I've been fighting the stomach flu for the last few days, and last night I finally had enough and went to the ER. They gave my some IV fluids, some medications for nausea and vomiting, and then I felt better so they sent me home. Now the whole right side of my face and neck feels really weird and tight. Do you have any idea what this could be?"

"I have my suspicions," I responded thoughtfully. "Do you know what medication they gave you for the nausea and vomiting last night?"

"Sorry, I guess I felt so lousy then that I really wasn't paying attention."

"That's OK, Margaret, we'll get a copy of the ER report faxed over right away." At that time, electronic records had not been developed, so many reports had to be transmitted by fax before they ended up in a paper chart.

Margaret had such a dramatic, unusual tightening of the right side of her face and neck areas to the point that she could not turn her head. Her neurological exam was otherwise normal, making a stroke or a serious central nervous system event less likely. She had all of the makings of an acute dystonic reaction most likely from an anti-nausea medication. The freshly acquired ER medication record gave up the last piece of the puzzle: *Compazine!* Compazine has traditionally been a common medication utilized to treat acute nausea and vomiting, but one of the significant side effects is acute spasms and dystonia. Margaret was urgently treated with an intramuscular dose of diphenhydramine, commonly known as Benadryl.

Five minutes later, I asked my nurse, "Can you please check up on Margaret and see if she is better?"

She appeared flummoxed. "Dr. Rowe, I just gave the Benadryl a few minutes ago."

I smiled with confidence, as if I was hiding a grand secret. "Just do me a favor and check, please."

She returned to me a few moments later, astonished. "I can't believe it . . . the spasms have completely disappeared!"

In dramatic fashion the troubling right-sided head and neck tightness had definitively resolved. The rapidity of normalization, while not clinically unexpected, is always captivating. I discharged a grateful Margaret home on scheduled Benadryl for the next forty-eight hours. Her now-rectified and beautiful smile was a satisfying result for both doctor and patient. It is always rewarding to possess the poise and experience to assist people in acute atypical crises.

It was Thursday a.m., and as a third-year medical student I nervously arrived on the hematology-oncology unit for another day of education and training. I had spent the last night reading up on chronic myelocytic leukemia (CML), and an overview of the procedure for performing a bone marrow biopsy. The interns, residents and students rotated for the privilege and opportunity of performing this test. In that era, bone marrow biopsy was performed bedside, and only with a local anesthetic, primitive compared to the more sophisticated sedation techniques used today. As the medical trainee completed the biopsy activity, all of the fellow medical students, staff and attending would watch in order to learn more about the technique, to be more prepared when their turn arrived, and to provide feedback to the student for improvement.

This day my number was up, and I was keenly aware of the level of expectations of dexterity and professionalism that I would soon be encountering. I felt prepared based on my reading and observing others completing the procedure; however, I also reminded myself of my neophyte status, and hoped that my performance would match the gravity of the moment. After morning rounds were completed, the team gathered in the patient's room for the minor intervention.

My blessed patient was Emmet Jasper, a rough-around-the-edges, yet good-hearted gentleman suffering from the aforementioned CML diagnosis. Emmet was a retired colonel in the United States Marine Corps. He exuded confidence, pride and an unshakable will to free himself from the ever-threatening tentacles of his blood malignancy. Despite appropriate chemotherapy measures and approaches, Mr. Jasper's blood counts did not seem to be recovering appropriately. Thus a bone marrow biopsy was required to ascertain what was occurring in the cellular level of blood cell production.

After I introduced Emmet to the team in attendance, we completed the positioning and instrument setup for the procedure. We had him lie facedown, and with a felt-tip pen I made a small mark over the posterior iliac crest of the right hip area. After cleaning the area with the antiseptic Betadine and deadening the area with local anesthetic, it was time to begin. I made a small nick in the skin, then firmly placed a T-shaped instrument called a trochar over the surface of the pelvic bone. Using a grinding, screwing motion similar to a corkscrew on a wine bottle, I felt the solid bony barrier gradually weaken; then with a telltale sign, a sickening crunch of the bone giving way and the instrument lurching forward and downward—I was now within the bone marrow. I used a syringe to draw up some of the marrow, and then with the trochar removed a core of bony tissue and its surrounding collection of blood mass to send to the pathologist. In a blink of an eye, the entire process effortlessly arrived at its inevitable conclusion. It had all progressed according to plan—we had gotten all of the biopsy and tissues that we needed, and Mr. Jasper seemed comfortable the entire time.

As I was getting ready to remove the biopsy apparatus and complete the procedure, I suddenly noticed something strange. Diffusely and from an unclear source in the room emanated a slight humming or buzzing noise. It began subtly, then progressively the eerie tone picked up in amplitude, pitch and timbre so that the entire room of students could hear it. I checked the TV and monitors, thinking it might be some type of electrical interference. As I was metaphorically scratching my head in an attempt to figure out the answer, a couple of my classmates burst out laughing, which spread around the entire team at lightning speed. At that instant I recognized the common biological source of the sound and its implications: Mr. Jasper had fallen asleep and was snoring! The weird rumbling nasal noises were icing on the cake, testifying to his level of relaxation and comfort. I was fortunate that he was making me look so good today: excellent level of anesthesia, successful bone marrow biopsy, no complications.

Midway through my final year of residency, I was serving as the chief on the inevitably busy internal medicine service. One weekend, Loretta Pfeiffer came in through the ER, reporting generalized body aches and fevers for the last several days. When I arrived in the department, she looked febrile and uncomfortable. I reviewed her vitals: Temperature of 104.0 F, pulse elevated at 120 beats per minute, BP stable at 130/85. Clearly, Loretta was acutely ill, most likely related to an infectious cause.

"Hi Loretta, when did you start feeling this way?" I asked.

"About four days ago. I started with a lot of body aches, then the fevers kicked in. Every four to six hours I get really flushed, break out in a sweat, then the chills come. It's absolutely miserable for me."

"Any cough, congestion, ear or sinus pain, pain with urination?"

"No Doc, none of those, just the fevers and body aches. Oh, and by the way, I just got back from vacation about ten days ago."

"Oh really? Where did you visit?"

"Honduras—we were working on a medical mission there for a week."

"OK, thanks for letting me know that." I nonchalantly made a note of that historical information, failing to recognize its potentially looming clinical significance.

As I progressed in my evaluation of Loretta, her findings, or rather lack of findings, became challenging and problematic. She had no evidence of an ear infection, pharyngitis, meningitis, and her lungs sounded clear. No abdominal or flank pain was present on exam. I received no reprieve from my dilemma on my labs and diagnostics either. Her blood count showed only a slightly elevated white blood cell count, urinalysis was unremarkable, and her flu testing was negative. The chest X-ray also did not display an obvious pneumonia, but I convinced myself of a possible early infiltrate in the right lower lobe, so I used pneumonia as a preliminary diagnosis. The lack of concordance between the severity of her fever and muscle pains versus her seemingly normal labs findings should have been a red flag. As evening approached, I admitted Loretta to the medical floor and placed her on IV antibiotics designed to treat community-acquired pneumonia.

On morning rounds, not much had changed. She continued to spike fevers and shook uncontrollably with chills. Loretta visibly recoiled and twinged when I touched any of her major muscle groups. Reexamination of her lungs, abdomen, ears, throat and neck did not reveal a solution to the deepening diagnostic mystery.

"Good morning, Loretta. It doesn't appear we've made much progress overnight," I began.

"Yes, that's an understatement. I would've believed that with all of the antibiotics and fluids I'd be feeling much better by now."

"I know, I agree with you. I'm calling in an infectious diseases consult and see if she can give us some further guidance. So sorry you are not improving yet."

"Thanks Dr. Rowe, please just get me better as fast as possible."

"Will do, Loretta, hope that today is the day." I attempted to project an outward sunny clinical confidence, but internally anguished under a gray cloud of discouragement. I had no idea what was going on with my patient. It appeared to be infectious, but after a complete inpatient day I was no closer to solving my clinical puzzle. I quietly slumped over the desk to write my notes for the morning, head spinning and attempting to gain a foothold on a list of elusive potential differential diagnoses.

Almost like divine intervention, a lifeline arrived unexpectedly from a phone call. The unit clerk picked up the phone and crisply answered, "Three West this is Susan, how can I help you . . .

Oh yes, Dr. Rowe is right here, I will have him speak with you right away. Dr. Rowe, hematology lab on line 2."

Almost comically interested and intrigued, I picked up the phone. "Dr. Rowe here."

"Hey Bruce, it's Michael down in hematology lab. You know that lady, Pfeiffer?"

"Yes, all too well I'm afraid; she is sick, febrile, and for the life of me I can't figure out why."

"Well, I think I've got your answer. Her white blood cell differential seemed a little bit weird, so I made a blood smear and looked at it under the microscope. She has a ton of microscopic protozoa on her peripheral smear . . . appears that it may be malaria. Any recent travel?"

"Yes—actually she just got back from Honduras a week and a half ago," I replied sheepishly. "Thanks a ton, Mike, you just cracked the code and cured our patient."

"Anytime, Bruce, you know that." The call abruptly terminated.

I hung up the phone, rubbed my temples, and resumed charting on my roster of patients, kicking myself for the delay in diagnosis. The small tidbit of clinical information, *the travel history to Honduras*, was the lynchpin in identifying malaria as the culprit. Minimizing the significance of Loretta's travel experience postponed appropriate therapy for nearly twenty-four hours. From that point forward, all of my patients admitted to the hospital have been asked about their travel history. Loretta was started on an appropriate antimalarial, and made a complete recovery without any long-term complications.

The fall of my senior year of high school arrived, and finally I felt like I was getting my bearings on the social spectrum of high school. Our cross country team was having a successful season, so my athletic prowess was garnering me some respect from some of my more popular and skeptical classmates. Homecoming was approaching, and my friend Emily met me in the hallway, needing to ask me something. I had a secret crush on her, so I hoped she was turning the tables on me to invite me to the homecoming dance.

"Hey Bruce, can I talk to you for a second?"

"Sure Emily, what's up?" trying to conceal my increasing optimism.

"Well Bruce, you know we have the big homecoming week coming up, and I was wondering . . ."

"Yes, Emily?" *This was it, get ready for the best homecoming ever in 3 . . . 2 . . . 1 . . .*

"Would you be able to volunteer for the Powder Puff game?" This was an unusual sporting event in which the senior girls split up into two teams and played a game of flag football in the stadium. Girls looked forward to the event for years.

"Oh . . . yeah . . . sure, I guess." *Man, I really thought I had broken through and snared the big prize.* "What do you need me to do for it?"

"We'd like you and some of your friends to serve as our cheerleaders."

Oh no! Traditionally a group of guys would dress up like female cheerleaders, the entire drag ensemble: makeup, pleated skirts, saddle shoes, even fake bosoms. I felt more than a little bit of discomfort with this proposal. It had taken me years to climb the social strata into a middling level of respectability, and I didn't want to squander it on a frivolous goofy event during homecoming week. Still, it has always been difficult for me to resist a pretty face, and I couldn't believe what I said next.

"OK Emily, my friends and I will do it for you guys."

"Thanks Bruce, looking forward to it!" She smiled in that incredibly wholesome, Midwestern manner, and departed.

I thought my cross country teammates were going to be furious with me for pulling them into this escapade. To my astonishment, they embraced the concept, their logic being that it would create exposure for our sports team and might even be fun. Reluctantly, I acquiesced, and soon it was the middle of homecoming week. On the asphalt track, my six buddies and I led the crowd in bawdy and silly cheers. My outfit consisted of a curly wig, overdone facial makeup, large balloon bosoms, a tight sweater and skirt ensemble and finally, the coup de grace, a pair of maroon tights. What I initially thought would be an awkward display was received as entertaining comedy by the crowd. My fellow cheerleaders and I poured on the humor and full-throated ironic yells.

I came to realize that it was OK for me to take chances and be weird in school; everything did not have to be controlled and scripted. To this day, when I return for my class reunions, invariably displayed is a yearbook picture of me in that crazy outfit, jumping up and down on the tarmac and lustily cheering on my team.

Whether a goofy outfit, an unusual case or a difficult patient, weirdness can be unsettling, pleasantly surprising or even humbling. It can rear its ugly head at remarkably unpredictable moments in medicine and life. My life and patient cases can always deviate from the expected trajectory, and although there is no magical formula, I need to be prepared and adaptable. In health care, the only sensible and pragmatic solution is to keep an open mind and consider all elements of information, no matter how seemingly trivial or atypical when caring for patients, normal or otherwise.

CHAPTER 17

MYOPIC

A tiny penny held up closely in front of an eye looms large enough to block out the entire view of the sun and the surrounding countryside. Similarly, an inappropriately narrow focus in approaches to a patient's medical care can result in shortfalls ranging from a frustrating disservice to life-threatening complications. Usually gracefully, but with occasional ham-handedness, I have juggled the rival demands of timely efficiency with patient thoroughness. Clinicians who prematurely winnow down to simplistic diagnoses may encounter an incorrect medical conclusion which could be detrimental to patients.

Colleen Feeney was a pleasant, elderly Catholic nun who I met as a resident on the inpatient medicine service at Waukesha Memorial Hospital. She had been vacationing with her brother, seeing multiple religious sites in Wisconsin before returning home to her native Michigan. Her trip was interrupted by an abrupt onset of an acute illness, manifested by fever to 102 degrees, chills, a moderately productive cough and wheezing. A chest

Xray performed in the ER readily revealed what appeared to be the culprit: a hazy left lower lung lobe infiltrate consistent with a community-acquired pneumonia. I admitted her to the medical floor and started her on antibiotics consisting of cefuroxime and erythromycin, standard antibiotic coverage for uncomplicated pneumonia back in the day. By this stage in residency I had developed a fair amount of confidence in treating patients for pneumonia, and I anticipated that Colleen's hospitalization would be routine. Within the next two to three days her condition would dramatically improve, and her brother would drive back from Michigan to pick her up.

Unfortunately, Sister Feeney's pneumonia ignored convention and was not improving as expected. Her fevers the following day had only decreased slightly to 101 degrees, and her chest X-ray actually looked a little bit worse compared to her admission film. On morning rounds, I led my team in the initial assessment and discussion.

"So, Sister Feeney, still not noticing much improvement compared to yesterday?"

"No, not really. I feel so wore out, still having fevers and chills, and coughing up a lot of mucus. I also found out my brother in Michigan is sick with a bad cold too. He's going to see the doctor today."

"Thanks for the info, Sister. We'll keep you on the antibiotics, IV fluids and breathing treatments for now. I believe you'll be feeling much better within the next forty-eight hours."

"Well I certainly hope so, Doctor, because right now I feel like I'm in some sort of weird holding pattern."

"Yes I agree—we'll touch base tomorrow, OK?"

"Sure Doctor, thanks," and turning to the medical entourage, she said, "God bless all of you fine doctors."

The following forty-eight hours did not progress according to plan. Colleen continued to have low-grade fevers and continued symptoms of pneumonia, with minimal improvement. My attending and I were scratching our heads at that point when, like a cataclysmic lightning bolt, a disturbing piece of medical information was revealed.

Colleen's nurse approached me at the nursing station prior to rounds. She appeared pained, like she had just learned some tragic news.

"Dr. Rowe?" she asked discretely.

"Yes Darcy, what's up?"

"I'm afraid that I have some bad news about Sister Colleen's family. Her brother just died from pneumonia yesterday."

In an instant, all of the confidence I possessed about treating inpatient pneumonia disappeared. My heart ached for Sister Colleen, who not only was struggling to get well but now was also saddled with the grief associated with suddenly losing her brother. Clearly, her pneumonia was unusual, and generally this meant either a viral or an atypical bacterial cause. Embarrassed at my overconfidence and clinical nearsightedness, my team and I raced to figure out an alternative pneumonia causation. We rapidly transferred Colleen to the ICU for continued care. Her testing did not indicate influenza, but a follow-up urine test did yield the culprit—an atypical bacterial infection known as Legionnaires' disease. Most likely she and her brother contracted the illness from a contaminated air conditioner water source in one of their hotel rooms on their travels. After she had a central venous line placed, high-dose antibiotics were administered. She made a full physical recovery, but on her discharge day I felt guilty that we didn't figure out her atypical pneumonia sooner. Perhaps we could have used the information from a prompt diagnosis of her illness to save her brother, instead of her brother's untimely death serving as the urgent impetus to rescue her.

Thomas Allen was a forty-two-year-old African American gentleman who had been a patient in my practice for several years, with a young and growing family. He was proud of having completed his MBA, taking evening classes while working on a full-time basis. He was engaging, goal-driven and always carried a book about motivational business with him. At this particular visit, however, Thomas seemed concerned. The normal radiant and bright white smile was missing from his countenance. His vocal delivery was stressed, conveying a preoccupation with some undisclosed weighty medical or emotional issue.

"Hi Tom," I quipped cheerfully, "how are things going for you these days?"

"I'm not sure, Doc, I just feel a little lightheaded, on edge, like my heart is racing, an anxious feeling really."

"How long have you noticed this?"

"About three to four weeks."

"Is it getting better, worse or staying about the same?"

"About the same, maybe a little worse."

"Any chest pain, shortness of breath, leg swelling, wheezing, sweats or fainting episodes?"

"Not really, but when we were driving over a long bridge in St. Louis last week I felt palpitations, nervous and on edge."

"Well, Tom, it sounds like you may have some anxiety and panic issues, and we can treat this problem with a medication called Paxil, which will prevent further anxiety episodes."

Tom's face asymmetrically squinted upward and twisted, to indicate a generous degree of skepticism with my preliminary assessment. "I'm not sure if that's it . . . I worry that it could be something more serious, maybe with my heart . . . I don't know what, just can't put my finger on it."

"That's understandable; let's examine you and see if we need to do any labs and testing to figure out your problem." My initial expectation was that his physical examination would prove to be unremarkable. Upon listening to his heart, however, my preconceived notions about Mr. Allen's physical health disintegrated. My stethoscope picked up a peculiarly irregular rhythm, not classical like atrial fibrillation, but something that I had never quite heard before. There were numerous premature-sounding beats, but they sounded like they were originating from multiple areas around the heart, and with a completely unpredictable pattern. Concerned, I completed a 12-lead ECG which showed very bizarre electrical wave complexes, out of sync and with multiple apparent lengths, duration, rhythms and morphologies. This finding was a double-edged sword: The ECG confirmed a cardiac diagnosis, but the mystery of what was causing the rhythm disturbance deepened and became more foreboding. *Bundle branch block? Congestive heart failure? Atrial fibrillation with aberrancy?*

I castigated myself for my shortsightedness in rushing to a mental health diagnosis before examining the patient. Chastened and armed with this new component of disturbing clinical information, I returned to the patient's room to formulate a new treatment plan.

"Tom, it looks like something unusual *is* occurring with your heart right now. The rhythm pattern and the appearance of the ECG is peculiar, and I honestly don't know what to make of it. We need to have you hospitalized immediately to identify the problem."

Mr. Allen straightened up slightly, attempting to hide a rising level of apprehension. "Oh . . . gee, I thought there might be a problem, but I didn't believe that it would be that big of a deal. Whatever you say, Dr. Rowe, let's figure it out."

Tom was promptly admitted to the hospital and seen by our cardiologist Dr. Rubin. An ultrasound of the heart called an echocardiogram showed a significant impairment of the efficiency of the heart; normally this should register at 65–70 percent, but his was alarmingly low at 20 percent. A workup for the cause of this dysfunction showed it to be either an unknown injury to the heart muscle, called idiopathic cardiomyopathy, or an infiltration of inflammatory material into the cardiac muscle, called sarcoidosis. He required an internal implantable cardiac defibrillator for arrhythmia protection and has gone on to live a normal, healthy life.

I was haunted by what could have occurred if I had simply completely brushed off Mr. Allen's concerns and reflexively treated him for a presumptive anxiety disorder. From this experience I promised myself not to be clinically nearsighted, and to avoid prejudging people and situations in medical practice until I had "the full story."

As I walked the short one-block journey from the high school to my home in the slanting rays of an unseasonably warm September afternoon, I thought about the next day's all-important cross country meet. It would be my final home invitational race as a high school senior, with twelve teams from all over southeastern Iowa participating. Our team had performed admirably up to this midpoint in the season, but all seven varsity runners had not achieved their absolute best simultaneously. I nervously contemplated the significance of the race tomorrow, and desperately wanted to close the curtain with our home course on a glorious, memorable high note. My teammates and I had completed a quality week of practice and were ready for the opportunity to prove ourselves on the hilly course. I entered the front door into our home, and as I set down my backpack, I felt a slight twinge of pain on my left outer chest wall area. *Probably nothing,* I casually contemplated.

Later in the evening, while navigating through my standard gauntlet of homework, I noticed that the pain on my left side was not ebbing away; in fact, it was subversively worsening, becoming more nagging and insistent. Ninety minutes later, the pain had become a significant negative force. I alternately felt feverish and chilled, and the chest pain was sharp, stabbing and flared up with even minimal inspirations. Turning my chest and attempting to lay flat on my back were incredibly painful maneuvers.

The untimely and disconcerting crescendo in the menacing pain caught me completely off guard. My thoughts turned to the upcoming important race and whether I would still be able to participate. *What's happening to me tonight? How can I run like this when every deep breath and movement feels like sheer torture?*

I knew that I had not sustained any trauma to the area and had eased up on the intensity of our training runs leading up to this crucial competition.

In my moment of discouragement, I tracked down one of my dad's old medical textbooks from his Navy days, and attempted to identify a reasonable medical explanation. Following ten minutes of symptom sleuthing, I figured out a provisional diagnosis: *pleurisy*. Patients with pleurisy have an inflammation of the chest wall lining, where the outer lung moves up and down along the inner layers of the chest cavity. Normally, this mobile interaction is smooth and uneventful; however, in the setting of pleurisy, viral-induced inflammation of the highly innervated membranes of the chest produce significant sharp pain with every breath. But come tomorrow, I wasn't simply going to be breathing at a baseline level of rest. For two miles and eleven minutes I would be running over irregular, hilly terrain, and attempting to oxygenate my system at a maximal respiratory rate and volume. The timing for this acute health malady could not have been any worse. I took four ibuprofen, placed a warm pack on my side, and turned in early, hoping for some respite from the pain in the a.m.

Morning inevitably arrived too soon, and unfortunately the demanding side affliction had not abated one iota. I resigned to myself that I would be forced to compete with a significant acute medical handicap. I attended my classes throughout the day with a sense of anger and frustration. My cross country swan song would thoroughly test my resolve to compete, with significant pain permeating every breath that I would take on the course.

Lake Keomah State Park was the naturalistic setting where we had run and competed countless times for training and meets. At least the weather cooperated—clear, pleasantly cool, low humidity, a dream late-afternoon day for a race while the fall equinox loomed for the following week. A low-hanging sun radiated filtered warmth through the nearby forest. My teammates and I changed into our running shoes, pinned our racing numbers to the front of our maroon-and-white singlets, and completed our warm-ups. It was game time, and we were ready. The starter called all of the teams to the starting line, a wide stretch of asphalt in front of the main lodge. It was a technicolor gathering of multiple teams and colors, complementing the early yellows and oranges emerging on the sprawling oak and maple trees which overhung and lined the road.

"Runners to your marks . . . Set!" The terse commands were followed by the startling, unceremonious crackle of the starter's pistol and a brief plume of ghostly white smoke. In a disconcerting instant we were off and running. The amorphous 140+ legged mass of humanity lurched forward, partly in unison, somewhat amoeba-like down the black-paved lane. With competitive efficiency, the running peloton lined up shoulder to shoulder and promptly filled every space on the roadway. After a quarter mile down the road the pack steadily elongated and thinned in width before turning and heading downhill onto a narrower gravel trail. My strategy was to initially conserve energy and avoid irritating my nagging chest problem. Throughout the first half of the race the relentless sorting of abilities continued, as I passed slower runners and still others mercilessly flashed by me. I was determined to simply run my race and make my move at an opportune time.

Along the picturesque lakeside the trail gracefully wound along the trees and shoreline filled with scattered clumps of runners. I passed the beach area, then the gravel pathway arched upward through the trees and past the campgrounds. With every stride the sharp needlelike daggers of pain mercilessly drove their tentacles into my left flank area. Past the campground, I allowed gravity to gently pull me down the long downhill. The race was nearing its exciting conclusion—one more steep hill to traverse, then a third of a mile straightaway back to the lodge to complete and close the loop.

At that moment, I briefly had thoughts of giving up. *This was so hard and painful, and really it was just one race, wasn't it?* Except that thinking was so shortsighted, and so much more was at stake. I needed to be able to persevere through incredible pain, come through for my teammates and hold myself accountable. Passing through the nadir of the valley and turning toward the final climb, I felt an inner flame ignite and a powerful voice emanate from my internal spirit. *This is your moment . . . give it your all . . . the time is now . . . pain is temporary . . . glory is forever!*

Out of nowhere, I dipped into my mental reserves to find the strength to banish the nagging pain far away from my consciousness and gradually began to increase my speed. I accelerated the intensity and rapidity of my cadence, and thunderously crested the hill. Swinging wide onto the main road back home I perceived a gentle, steady cooling breeze lovingly press against my backside. My confidence was surging, endorphins repelling the nociceptive impulses from my adrenaline-immersed brain. Like a farmer engaging in a bountiful harvest, scythe-like I methodically picked off several ripe and vulnerable runners, continuously improving my placing on the straightaway bound for the finish line.

It was a trying, brutal experience, but served as a moment of pride that I conquered the internal demons of pain and voices of self-doubt. A few agonizing minutes later, clutching my side and close to tears, I crossed the finish line into the flag-draped chute. *Not bad . . . seventh place, second-best time on my team.* Now the waiting game began to see how my five other teammates finished behind me, and where our team would ultimately place. I found the nearest tall white oak tree and leaned my back against it, completely spent from the Herculean effort. Gradually the course emptied itself of all of the remaining harriers, and the tabulations began in earnest. Conversing with my teammates, it became clear that everyone had run their best race.

A few minutes later, Coach Van Allen came over to our team circle. "Congrats boys, you won your home meet . . . by one point!"

An outburst of high fives and whoops joyfully erupted from our group. Although my ever-present chest wall pain kept my celebration muted, I was delighted that we were successful as a team, and my ability to push through a short-term setback contributed to our victory.

Stephen Morris was a wonderful, talented fifty-three-year-old African American gentleman whom I had known in clinical practice for the last several years. He was always immaculately dressed, had a professorial bearing, with a keen business and financial mind. We both possessed a dry sense of humor, and our visits were rich with satire and terrible puns. A few years ago Stephen began struggling with some intermittent lower back pain.

"Hi Stephen, what's up with your back?" I asked.

"Well, it's kind of weird, Dr. Rowe. Some days it's really stiff in my lower back, and it takes awhile to get the kinks out. Once I get moving it seems to be fine. I'm bothered because it's happening more frequently now. Maybe I need some physical therapy or something."

"Yes, PT often does the trick. Maybe you have a bit of early arthritis settling in your lumbar spine. Let's take a look at things and figure out what we should do next."

Stephen's back exam was generally negative except for some mild stiffness, which could be on account of muscle spasms or degenerative changes of the lower spine. There were no signs of a vertebral fracture or sciatica. X-rays of the lumbar spine were negative except for findings of sacroileitis, an inflammation where the back joins the pelvis. At the time this appeared to be an incidental finding, but it would come back later to haunt me. I prescribed him an anti-inflammatory and some muscle relaxants and referred him to the physical therapist. He followed up with me in the office several weeks later.

"I thought you fixed my back for a little while there Doc, but now that same stiffness and pain is back again!"

"Man, that stinks, Mr. Morris. Fortunately your back exam is reassuring for now. Let's get back to PT again for some more sessions and keep me updated."

"Alright Dr. Rowe, let's try 'er again."

Unfortunately, the therapy sessions did not result in long-term benefit. Every few months like clockwork Stephen would return with the recurrent problem of low back pain, and the more operative word *stiffness*. After exchanging our usual pleasantries and jokes, I would reiterate the usual treatment plan.

A few months later, Mr. Morris presented to a chiropractor's office for a second opinion. Follow-up spinal X-rays obtained two years after our initial films confirmed the diagnosis that I should have made earlier in the process: a ridged, bamboo-like appearance of the spine, consistent with an autoimmune inflammatory disease called ankylosing spondylitis (AS). A subsequent blood test in our office confirmed a positive HLA—B27 level consistent with AS. The subtle finding on the initial lumbar X-ray and the overriding concern of stiffness should have been a tip-off that this was an inflammatory process and not the garden variety wear and tear osteoarthritis. Because of this inflammatory spinal disease, the PT and medications that I had repetitively employed for him would never work for long.

My diagnostic approach to Stephen proved to be myopic, related to a combination of excessive socialization during visits and clinging to a diagnosis of degenerative arthritis and muscle spasm long after facts of the case proved otherwise. After a referral to a rheumatologist and a pharmaceutical regimen of powerful anti-inflammatories and immune-modulating agents, Stephen is living a full and productive life. His case story serves as a constant reminder to me to maintain an appropriate focus on the patient's clinical story, and to avoid being shortsighted with limited common diagnoses or distracting social banter.

Despite my best efforts and trying to be a good assistant, I could never get off on the right foot with Dr. Simmons. He was one of the obstetrical attending physicians who mentored me during my residency training. Whenever his patients arrived on the unit, I promptly evaluated them, called him with regular updates, and maintained an excruciating level of attention and detail caring for his expectant mothers. Finally, when the moment of truth arrived for the delivery, he would gently nudge me out of the way and complete the delivery himself. I became progressively disillusioned and frustrated by the entire process. *Why bother? He's just gonna swoop in and do the whole thing himself and leave me out in the cold.* Fortunately, I possessed too much pride and dedication to the patients to abandon my responsibilities that easily. For weeks, the same process continued unabated—my involvement in the final stages of delivery remained minimal, and I was relegated to being a glorified assistant.

Exasperated, I vented my frustrations in private to Ryan, my senior resident who split call with me.

"Ry—this really sucks . . . Simmons doesn't let me do jack, I work hard for him all day and then when the moment of truth arrives, I'm just a spectator."

Ryan gave me a knowing smile and regarded me with reassurance. "Sometimes, Bruce, you just gotta be patient and let things play themselves out."

"Alright, I'll keep trying, I hate just standing there like a dope during the delivery."

"Maybe 'cause you're just 'standing there,' he's not comfortable letting you do anything."

Touché. Perhaps my negative attitude was on display when Dr. Simmons and I were working together. I made a priority of being the best damn assistant ever with him going forward—handing him instruments, prepping for the delivery, cleaning up afterwards, everything. I needed to let go of the myopic view of not doing anything and embrace observational learning for now. Hopefully soon I would get my chance. A week later, Ryan had a subtle message for me from Dr. Simmons.

"Hey—Simmons says you gotta be patient with doing deliveries, he's gotta get comfortable with you, then you'll get your chance, alright?"

I appreciated that Ryan had laid some positive groundwork for me. "Thanks Ryan, I'll dial it back a little, and take things as they come."

A few typical Simmons deliveries later, my opportunity arrived. Our lady had been pushing for about an hour and was imminently ready to deliver. Doc Simmons and I gowned up together, but instead of purposely standing in front of me this time, we stood abreast of each other.

"OK Bruce . . . I'm going to help you through this one. Let's take our time through this process, the baby looks fine on the monitor."

"Thanks Dr. Simmons, whatever you say."

Shortly thereafter, the infant's head stretched the outer vaginal tissues, making ready its plan to emerge into the world. This is where Dr. Simmons' sense of patience and timing really showed through.

"Now, the baby is slowly extending the perineum. It would be tempting to have her push quickly and get this baby delivered immediately. However, that would risk causing a lot of trauma, tears and tissue damage. Baby looks fine on the monitor. Slow and steady wins the race, got it?"

"Yes, that's really good advice, thanks."

He placed his hands over mine, and for every contraction and outward movement of the infant's head, he had me apply gentle counterpressure to keep the delivery process orderly and controlled. Our mom-to-be had excellent pain control with her epidural anesthesia, so we were not prolonging any agony. Dr. Simmons gently kept his hands cupped over mine, allowing me to actively control the delivery, but ready to take over at a moment's notice. It was a simultaneously awkward and reassuring medical choreography. Over the next several contractions, the baby's head progressively increased its outward appearance. Finally, baby Alex was born, beautiful and healthy on all accounts.

"See there Bruce? Look at that perineum! That's what an orderly, controlled childbirth gets you! Only a few small labial and vaginal abrasions, nothing that even needs stitches! You rush that delivery, and you could end up with a third- or fourth-degree tear, which is a lot of trauma and recovery time. Pretty neat huh?"

"Why yes, absolutely." Humbled and ashamed at my nearsighted impatience, I realized that I had focused more on the delivery process as opposed to learning to perfect my overall medical craft. Dr. Simmons seemed unconventional and peculiar at times with his approaches. However, I gained powerful insight that becoming a talented physician not only involves increasing knowledge and perfecting technical expertise, but also cultivating a kind and patient heart.

CHAPTER 18

MAGIC

Springtime came early, just in time for the track season to begin for my senior year in high school. The third Saturday in April finally arrived, and the Osky Relays were set for another historic running, poised to add yet another chapter to its illustrious history. On race day, dawn was slightly chilly, but rapidly warmed up to the mid-70s by early afternoon. Puffy cumulus clouds scuttled by quickly, then progressively thinned and ultimately disappeared, leaving a vast azure expanse of sky to greet the multitude of track and field competitors. Sunshine beamed on the athletes and fans alike, at a higher angle and with shorter shadows, foreshadowing longer and warmer days to come. Twenty competing teams from all over the central and southeast Iowa region combined in a kaleidoscopic splash of color. It was setting up to be a perfect day for athletic pursuits.

Up to that point, I had produced a fairly successful running season. My list of competitive events included the individual 800-meter, 1600-meter, 3200-meter runs as well as the 4 x 800-meter relay. I had never finished worse than third place in any of my races that spring. The current track season was shaping up for a momentous conclusion. All of my off-season work was paying big dividends and culminating with a degree of athleticism that I had only dreamed of as a clumsy middle schooler. Instead of sitting on the bench, sidelines or stands watching the physical exploits of my more talented brethren, this time I was the focus of attention.

Time was running out to qualify for the prestigious Drake Relays and the Iowa High School Track and Field Championships in Des Moines. As I warmed up on the back stretch of my home track, my mind reflected on all of the effort that went into getting to this level. Hundreds of miles of long summer runs on country gravel roads, leading our cross country team to several fall meet victories, winter months lifting weights and improving core strength, early spring races, all pointed to this exact moment. I felt a mixture of pride and trepidation this day, with some twinges of pressure and weighty expectations to come through in my slate of events.

Throughout my entire track career, my favorite of all events in which to compete was the 1600-meter run. It is the meter equivalent of the mile run, although in college and international competition the 1500-meter distance is considered the true "metric mile." Back then it usually took me around four minutes and forty seconds to complete the four full revolutions on the 400-meter track. For me, it is the pinnacle of true athleticism; you start the race, maintain a strong pace, and try to hold a rapid rate with your legs for as long as humanly possible. It is the ultimate, divine convergence of sprinting and endurance—you must have both skills, and cannot possess just one or the other.

Often the fourth lap becomes sheer torture, as you try to stave off your competitors and push the pace a little bit faster, while simultaneously feeling the burning, leaden feeling of lactic acid building up in your legs, begging for mercy and reprieve. This is the point when the contending runners, especially upperclassmen, often draw upon their levels of experience and mental fortitude to prevail over similar physically talented running competition.

It had been a good day so far—I had taken a respectable second place in the 800-meter event with a personal record time. I felt the time inexorably march by, and soon my marquee event approached. The announcements for first call, second call, final call for the 1600-meter run all came and went. I stripped off my sweat suit and looked down at my singlet emblazoned in maroon and white with a cursive upsloping script, "Osky," short for Oskaloosa, prominently gracing the front. My maroon shorts were silky smooth and felt aerodynamic. This would be the final time I would wear this uniform for a race on my home track. I attempted to blot out any nostalgia from my mind as I entered into my final race preparation.

My main competition today was an extremely talented junior competing for the Grinnell Tigers named Mark Brown. Mark had been my nemesis all season long—many of my second-place finishes this year had been at his expense. I had come close multiple times to beating him, but up until now had never able to accomplish that feat. Today, however, I liked my chances. I had a lot on the line in this race: a chance to run at the Drake Relays, improve my state qualifying time, make a good impression on my town, and represent my team with pride. Never in my life had I felt so physically and mentally prepared for a sports endeavor. Perhaps this was going to be the day which I had been waiting for my entire athletic life . . . a chance at local sports immortality and permanently etching my name in the pantheon of Oskaloosa High School sports heroes and legends. Just four minutes and change separated me from my destiny and the final answer.

The starter called all of us runners to the line. Obligingly we all scampered up to the white curvilinear arc which defined the starting line for the 1600-meter run. I was crouched forward in my starting stance, ready to charge forward, flanked by two of my teammates in Lane 3. Mark Brown was two lanes to my right in 5, staggered slightly in front of me. I fervently hoped that by race's end that would no longer be the case. "Runners to your marks!" belted out the starter, followed a moment later by "Set!" and then a pregnant pause, gun raised, and finally the crackle of the starter's pistol with a rapidly ejecting white plume of smoke.

Swiftly I responded to the start signal and rapidly maneuvered myself into a favorable position in about fourth or fifth place on the outside, good shape so far. Mark was on my right, slightly behind me. The lead runners set a good pace and we passed the halfway mark in about 2:18. This was a good sign—a strong pace, but not one that would be a killer in the end and cause the field to fade and collapse. One more revolution around the track, and as the final lap bell clanged, I heard the timer call out the split for the three-quarter mark—3:27! I had an opportunity to set another personal record, maybe qualify for the higher sports glory for which I had always dreamed. I was now in second, and as we rounded turn one, the echoes of the final bell reverberating in my consciousness, I let the adrenaline and centrifugal force swing me wide and pass the lead runner. *Glory! Honor! Pure joy!* I was in the lead in the marquee event of the entire meet, with more rewards surely in store.

As we rounded turn two into the backstretch, I heard the faster footfalls, the heavy breathing, the confident striding behind my immediate right, followed by the passage of an orange, white and black jersey. It was Mark Brown! He passed me speedily and settled in front of me comfortably as we rocketed along the backstretch. Previously, he would open up a big gap and coast to the finish; I was determined not to let this happen. I rapidly made up the difference and was immediately behind him now, holding fast. *I can do this! Today is going to be different!* We rounded turns three and four at dazzling speed. I had never felt so strong and mentally focused this late in a race, and now the crowd rose to its feet, sensing an epic finish. I pulled to the outside, and now was only a half a meter off of the lead. On the frontstretch, I implemented my final maneuver—a steady increase in speed every ten meters with the hopes of wearing Mark down and getting to the tape first.

Mark was having none of it. Being a master tactician and sterling athlete in his own right, he matched me stride for stride, and in the last twenty meters, brought forth a frenetic cadence that I simply could not match. He hit the tape about a half a second in front of me, once again besting me in our recurrent battle of legs and wills. The crowd roared its appreciation and approval, and my moderate disappointment with losing was mitigated by the response of the spectators and knowing that I gave it my all, and most likely set a personal record in my favorite event.

Mark and I exchanged tired congratulations, stood side by side for a few moments with our arms around each other, and then we departed for our respective teams and coaches.

But just how fast did I run today? Anxiously, I searched out the group of timers, my father among them, looking to lock on my designated timekeeper. My father brought over Charlie, one of the fellow timers, over to see me. They both exuded pride, beaming and grinning from ear to ear. Charlie held up the round blue plastic digital chronograph for me to see. *It read 4:34.1!* That was the fastest time in the 1600-meter that I had ever run, beating my previous best mark by over five seconds! In sheer delight, drenched in sweat, I wrapped my arms around them in a three-man embrace, and I heard the words every son wants to hear from his father, "Son . . . I'm so very proud of you!" Never in my life had finishing second felt so wonderful.

As it turned out, the times in the state were very competitive that year, and I missed qualifying for the Drake Relays and the state meet by less than a second. I never ran a 1600-meter race that fast again. But as sunset drew upon my scholastic track and field career, I never forgot that magical feeling of pride and accomplishment of running and performing at my absolute best for all to see.

On a few select occasions in a medical career, a patient comes into a doctor's life who seemingly defies all of the odds and recovers from a disease or situation that seemed unsurmountable. In retrospect, I found myself scratching my head attempting to formulate a hypothesis for exactly what had taken place, only to arrive at the identical conclusion every time: It was magical, mystical, a miracle as it were, with no logical explanation for the turn of events. Even though these patient scenarios meant that I was either wrong in my prognosis or had no role in the resolution of the medical problem, it was still a privilege to be a first-row witness to my patient's wondrous and joyous recovery.

Robert Kramer was in his mid-sixties when he presented to my office in the fall of my first year as practicing family physician. I was still a neophyte, fresh off the residency track where if I had questions or concerns about a patient, I would always run it past my superior attending physician. Now I was on my own, fledgling out of the nest, responsible for the health and well-being of many lives in my community. Robert was seeing me for the first time, and he generally appeared to be healthy. However, he was moderately overweight and smoked three-quarters to one pack of cigarettes per day. He was concerned about some new-onset fatigue and hoarseness.

"Mr. Kramer, when did you notice your hoarseness begin?"

"About six weeks ago, I guess."

"Any weight loss, shortness of breath or coughing up blood?"

"No, none of those."

"How tired have you been feeling?"

"A lot—I can't even do the fall leaf cleanup this year, like I usually do."

"How long have you been a smoker?"

"I don't know, maybe forty-five years."

"Are you coughing at all these days?"

"Yes, just a little, sometimes dry, occasionally wet, no blood though."

I ordered some labs and a chest X-ray, and although the labs would take a day or two to return, the X-ray image projected an unmistakable problem—a large 9 cm left upper lobe mass of the lung which was highly suspicious for a lung cancer. It could explain Mr. Kramer's weakness, persistent cough and hoarseness. For the first time as a young attending I had to complete one of the most difficult responsibilities in medicine: delivering bad news to a patient.

Outside Robert's room I screened the X-ray carefully once more to verify I had the correct information, knocked and, attempting to conceal my trepidation, opened the door. I sat down in my ubiquitous swiveling circular chair and turned to face Robert and his wife.

"Well, Mr. Kramer, I reviewed your chest X-ray, and there is a large mass in the lung which is very unusual and appears to be suspicious for cancer . . . I'm so sorry to have to tell you this." I showed him and his wife the X-ray film with the mass on it. It was angry, opaque and lobular, completely alien and out of place in contrast with normal dark tranquility of the appropriately aerated lung tissue. Since we did not yet have a biopsy result, I was careful not to pronounce with complete certainty that it was cancer, rather a strong suspicion. As I completed delivering this terrible news to him, I looked at the wall out of the corner of my eye and I captured a photo in a frame; it was my newborn daughter Allison, in a beautiful floral infant dress. The hopefulness of my daughter's new life represented a painful juxtaposition with my patient's new worrisome diagnosis.

The silence after I had finished my depressing soliloquy was palpable. Mrs. Kramer spoke first.

"I hope this wasn't anything I did wrong, I always tried to make healthy and nutritious meals for us."

"No, Mrs. Kramer, this isn't related to that. Most likely it's related to cigarette smoking and genetics."

Robert spoke through slightly moistened eyes. "Well Doc, thanks for figuring this out, even though I really don't like the possible result very much. What's next?"

I stared at him and his wife, already amazed at his stoicism and determination in the face of such bleak news. In my mind, I felt that his survival may be measured only in months, given the size and nature of the cancer. We did not discuss those potential implications today, as it could significantly discourage him and deprive him of any remaining shreds of hope.

"We'll need to get you set up for a biopsy, obtain some additional CT scans for staging purposes and, finally, an outstanding oncologist to manage your treatment."

OK Doc, sounds good, please help me get through this. Let's stay in close contact, alright?"

"Yes sir, I would like that idea very much." I was surprised that at this point I seemed more upset than he was, although I am certain that many tears were shed by Robert in the privacy of his own home and immediate family.

For the next few months, our interactions were more sporadic, given his need to have the oncology service be the primary driver of his care at that stage of his disease process. A bronchoscopy and biopsy confirmed a diagnosis of large cell lung cancer. The total body CT scan and bone scans presented us with the first elements of good news: Although the primary tumor was quite large, there was no evidence of metastasis (i.e., spread) to other areas of the body.

He began a course of chemotherapy and radiation, which obviously produced a significant amount of fatigue, weight decrease and hair loss. I saw him once during the middle of this process, and I was struck by the twinkle of his gray eyes piercing through the pale gloom and despair projected by his fragile frame. It was strange—his eyes radiated serenity, calmness, even confidence in the face of such overwhelmingly negative odds. His cancer was non-operable, and it was fairly well-established that people with lung cancer usually did not do very well long-term. Was there some insight or privileged information he knew that I did not? I wished him and his wife well. We optimistically planned a follow-up visit, although with all honesty I believed that that day could represent our last visit together,

Autumn arrived again, and lo and behold, Mr. Kramer was once again back in our office. He had completed his chemotherapy and radiation treatments, his thick shock of vibrant white hair had completely grown back, and his ruddy brown skin color had returned. Another bonus was that he had stopped smoking nine-plus months before. He looked well and he stated that he felt even better, perhaps the best he had in five years. His physical exam was reassuring that day, he had gained some weight back, and the last CT scan showed a shrinking tumor volume. The hoarseness of his voice had abated, and his fatigue was regressing. I was astonished at the turnaround and congratulated him on all of his accomplishments in the last year.

"Hey Robert . . . how about we recheck your chest X-ray today and see how things are progressing?"

Robert and his wife seemed intrigued, maybe even optimistic. "Yes, I'd like to know how we are doing."

Nervously, I sent him down for the chest imaging, and as I gingerly placed the radiographic film on the lightbox, I was stunned by what I saw . . . *nothing! Where did the tumor go?* Pleasantly bewildered, I checked the margin of the film to make sure that I had the chest film of the right person. *Yes—Robert Kramer!* I returned to the room and gave the Kramers the exciting and encouraging news, holding the now normal-appearing film up toward the fluorescent lighting.

"Mr. Kramer, I see absolutely no evidence that there is any residual tumor in the chest today. I cannot explain this by any other means than this is . . . a miracle!"

His eyes twinkled brighter than ever before, a broad smile and toothy grin emerged, and his body language and posture optimistically reached upward toward the heavens. "Really? I mean, you're shitting me, right? I just can't believe it!"

I cautiously replied, "Well, we should recheck the CT scan again now to confirm this, and you will need follow-up scans every three months for now, but at this point it looks like your cancer is in complete remission. At this point, you are officially designated my *Miracle Man!*"

Robert and his wife beamed and left the office with an unbelievable visual lightness of their feet, as if a year's worth of an awkward, leaden yoke of worry had been lifted from them. Subsequent medical evaluations and CT scans over the years continued to show him to be cancer-free; his lung cancer never returned again to torment his physical being and emotional psyche. For fifteen years, Robert lived a healthy, wonderful rewarding life before succumbing to an unrelated liver cancer in his mid-eighties. To this day, he remains a wonderful testament to the individual power of hope and faith when confronting a seemingly insurmountable physical illness. Enchanted miracles can and will happen to blessed patients in a medical practice.

Amanda Mueller was a delightful thirty-two-year-old white female, who had been my patient for the last several years. She had been happily married for the last six years, but despite their best efforts had not been able to successfully conceive a child. My heart ached for her and her husband, who had their hopes repeatedly dashed with multiple negative urine pregnancy tests in our office. Infertility workups were essentially inconclusive, and facing the emotionally challenging and financially daunting prospect of fertility specialists and IVF treatments, she and her husband elected to abandon their efforts at having biological children. Six months previously, they had adopted a wonderful baby boy who had brought them much joy in their lives. When we met for a follow-up office visit, I congratulated her on her adopted infant son. Seeing a bit of discouragement and sense of failure in her eyes, I offered emotional support to her.

"Listen Amanda, I know how much having a child of your own meant to you previously. I hope that you are happy and enjoying the gifts of your new baby."

"Thanks Dr. Rowe, I am thrilled to be a mother to little Nathan here right now. He is a beautiful gem and his father and I love him very much." She seemed comforted by my words of optimism and encouragement. We exchanged a warm embrace and made plans to see her for an annual physical in about six months.

Surprisingly, Amanda appeared on my schedule only three months later with a chief complaint of "missed periods." I emotionally prepared myself for our visit with some trepidation, not wanting to sow another layer of heartbreak on top of this sensitive issue.

"Hi Amanda, so you have been having irregular periods again?" I asked gently.

"Yes Doc, I haven't had a cycle for the last two months, no spotting or bleeding at all."

"Any bloating, breast tenderness, weight gain, nausea?"

"Yes, I've noticed all of those things off and on for the last few weeks," Amanda replied almost nonchalantly. When she had irregular menses previously, Amanda never indicated nausea or breast tenderness. I cautiously selected my word choices when reviewing the treatment plan with my vulnerable patient.

"I hate to say this, Amanda, but I really wonder if you could be pregnant. Hard as it is to believe, we should check a urine pregnancy test."

"Oh no, Dr. Rowe, please don't do this to me today . . . it upsets me just thinking about doing that test and always getting the same sad result. Is there something else we can check?"

I made a deal with Amanda. She agreed to go to the hospital and have her urine test and other blood work completed to avoid the negative flashbacks of our laboratory, followed by a return visit tomorrow. In the morning, I reviewed the results with her—a positive urine pregnancy test, and a serum quantitive pregnancy test which was also positive. Even with all of that encouraging data, I was careful in how I framed the news: I advised her that the pregnancy test was positive, not that she was pregnant. Heaven forbid that she had a blighted ovum, miscarriage or some other type of nonviable pregnancy, which would be the ultimate disappointment. Cautiously, she and her husband were elated with the unexpected news. Her early ultrasound confirmed a healthy, viable pregnancy, and thirty-eight weeks later she delivered a beautiful baby girl. Three years after that, they were again blessed with a naturally conceived healthy baby girl, making their family complete.

Why did Amanda dramatically achieve a pregnancy after years of trying and no optimistic signs that it would be possible? As with Robert's situation, I have no clear rational explanation. Sometime in discouraging medical situations with no resolution in sight, a magical moment may occur when it is least expected. I felt fortunate to witness such a wonderful and special moment in a young couple's life.

When I was in high school my father carried a buckeye with him in his pocket. He believed that it brought him good luck, and often he was proven correct. During my sophomore year the high school football team went undefeated. Invariably the buckeye was snugly and securely in his pocket when I won my first individual track race. With my poor natural athletic ability, I had never won anything sporting in my life. Upon graduation from medical school, I ceremoniously carried a buckeye from Laura's family home in rural Iowa in my front right pocket, a powerful symbolism to my father's memory that "we finally did it!" I always loved its beautiful simplicity—a smooth, beautiful oblate object, timeless and a representation of hopeful potential, with nurturing and time ultimately destined to become a towering, glorious shade tree.

A few years ago, the practice of medicine was becoming quite difficult and challenging. Patients were exceedingly complicated from a medical standpoint, family members were constantly unhappy, even registering baseless complaints about the quality of care that I was providing. Every day in the clinic was becoming a struggle; people became depersonalized objects, a perceived awful fifteen-minute obstacle to conquer and overcome. I had never felt this level of discouragement in my decade-plus years of medical practice. With every passing day and week, I began to feel a sense of despair about possibly losing my edge as a talented family physician.

In recent years, whenever I have struggled mightily with my depressive emotions, I engaged in a simple yet powerful ritual: I prayed specifically to my late father. Even though he had been gone nearly twenty-five years, I still felt his presence at times, especially during moments of significant emotional discouragement. During my noontime swim one day, I made a special appeal to Dad for a few moments on my breaststroke:

Dad, I know that you see everything going on in my life right now, and I've been struggling with it all recently. Please watch over me, and provide some hope and comfort to my family and me. I remain open to any sign of your presence. I love you and miss you always.

At the end of the clinic day, I picked up my daughter Julia from her dance class. The weather was unusually cool and crisp for a late September afternoon. When we arrived home, I wanted to do something athletic rather than simply going inside and powering down for the evening.

"Hey Juju, how about we go outside and play catch with the football for a little bit?" I hoped that a joyful activity with my daughter would take my mind off of the stressors of the workplace.

"Yeah Dad, sounds good, let's do it!"

For about twenty minutes we exchanged wobbly spirals back and forth between us, about thirty feet apart, enjoying the coolness of the early autumn afternoon and exchanging joyful banter about our respective days at work and school.

At that point, Julia ran to her right and tripped slightly over a small lump in the ground. She stopped to look at the obvious, awkward irregularity in the normally flat front yard of our home. Curiosity elevated, she kicked at the lump with her foot, and a solid brown nodule tumbled out and emerged to the surface.

"Hey Dad, what's this?"

It was a buckeye! I could not believe it. We don't even have an identifiable buckeye tree near our home, so it didn't fall from a local tree. The logical explanation is that an enterprising squirrel stashed it away in the ground recently in preparation for a long winter of foraging. My faith convinced me that it was my father getting the comforting message to me that in times of great difficulty, "everything will be OK." Even though I didn't have the gift of many years as I would have liked with my father, I have his inspiration and a constant spiritual sense of his presence every day. The glorious mysteries of life, whether a regressing cancer, unexpected pregnancy, or a divine reassurance, serve to maintain my hopefulness and joy and restore my faith in the sheer beauty of human existence.

CHAPTER 19

TWILIGHT

In the biomedical engineering world, the biological systems of the human body are analyzed in the prism of mechanical design and functionality. Having studied both engineering and medicine, I have realized that one prominent commonality between humans and machines is that both can wear out and break down. Doctors and engineers strive to maintain the health of the organism or the structural system. When failures occur, significant time and energy is placed into investigating "what went wrong," and how to prevent recurrent problems. Unfortunately, often people and machines inevitably fail completely, becoming so damaged that no well-intentioned intervention can rectify the problem. Whether a ninety-year-old patient at the end of life or a tragically sick newborn, having to tell a family "there is nothing else we can do" is one of the worst experiences in medicine. It is the mental balancing act of confronting defeat with a tacit acknowledgment of the impermanence of everyone's life.

The cradle-to-grave pathway of biological life is unpredictable and complicated. Through the years, some dying processes in my patients have been beautiful and graceful, an epitome of "going gently into that good night." Other human losses were shocking and unexpected, much like the Greek Fates with anxious scissors impulsively severing the life skein: a grandmother who committed suicide by running her car in an enclosed garage; a previously healthy fifty-five-year-old man who dropped dead of a heart attack while jogging; or a young partner struck dead walking his dog by a distressed driver having a medical emergency. Hospice teams have been my faithful companions for comforting patients and families through the heartbreaking process of saying goodbye. The specter of death is best approached with compassion and a degree of reverence for the sacredness of life.

My interesting and eccentric Great-grandmother Marintha died in 1975, when I was seven. She had been bedridden for many years due to a hip fracture that failed to heal properly, and my saintly Aunt Grace cared for her continuously until her passing. As we approached the rose-colored metallic casket, my father placed a comforting and reassuring hand on my slight, trembling frame.

"Bruce, why don't you gently touch her hand?" he asked quietly.

I tentatively palpated the pale white shriveled appendage. "It feels really cold," I answered quizzically.

"That's because her soul has escaped up into heaven."

"Is my soul going to run away up into heaven?" I asked with escalating panic.

His eyes twinkled. "Not anytime soon. You have to be old like Great-grandma Rowe."

I noticed that only the top half of her body was showing. "What happened to her legs?" I was more confused than ever. My first exposure to a funeral home experience was awkward, and I felt very out of place in this uncertain, somber environment.

My dad laughed softly. "Bruce, her legs are there! The lower half of the casket lid is closed because that is how we usually show people in the funeral home after they die . . . Hey Jerry," asking in a subtle voice to the funeral home director. "Can you show her lower legs for my son so that he understands?"

Jerry gave a warm smile. "Sure, no problem." He discreetly raised the right side half of the metallic lid to reveal an intact body and her rigid, atrophied lower extremities. My father and his friend framed a gloomy event in an lighthearted manner, and for me that was a blessing.

Peter Cantwell was a sixty-five-year-old white male who had been under my care for the last several years. Six months previously he had a complete physical and lab studies which were completely normal and reassuring. On a chilly windy day in late October, he presented to my clinic with a history of bright red blood in his urine which was clearly visible and painless. Unfortunately a CT scan confirmed a tumor in the right kidney which was highly suspicious for a malignancy. Soon thereafter he underwent surgical removal of the affected kidney, which confirmed a particularly virulent type of cancer called a small cell cancer; this type of cancer has a high likelihood to grow, metastasize, and fail to respond to conventional chemotherapy and radiation interventions. He was treated with both of these modalities after surgical removal, and the next several months were uneventful for any significant complications.

Approximately nine months postoperatively, Peter presented with increasing shortness of breath, cough productive of bloody sputum and fatigue. Repeat CT scan of the body showed spread of the cancer throughout the abdomen and into the lungs. He had a markedly elevated calcium level, which indicated extension of the tumor into bony structures. This foretold a very unfavorable clinical prognosis and limited prospects for survival. Presenting the bad news to Peter and his family was a necessary and unfortunate exercise. Every situation involving the presentation of an adverse medical report is unique and presents its own challenges. Peter's wife struggled mightily to maintain a façade of self-control over her fears and sadness.

Mr. Cantwell's subsequent clinical course remained unfavorable and progressive. His family sought out a second opinion from the local tertiary medical center, which confirmed his poor prognosis. He was placed into home hospice, where a few weeks later I was contacted by his daughter, a triage nurse in my clinic and a family friend—he was entering an active dying process, and I left clinic immediately to go see him. Unfortunately, he had passed away before I could make it to his home.

After a final outpouring of tears and heartfelt embraces, almost on cue the cooks who worked at his family's restaurant brought over food for a late dinner. As we ate the welcome meal, I glanced through the archway at Peter's lifeless body, slumping in the distance of the front living room. It was a surreal scene, but the moment felt appropriate—savoring an intimate dining experience, lives moving forward, respectful laughter and conversation. Finally the tribulations that formed the epilogue of a glorious life had arrived at a merciful end.

The "bad news" encounters and sad interactions I have had with my patients over the years have been fascinating in terms of their complexity and emotional depth. Most medical school graduates in my era did not have significant training in delivering serious, ominous medical results to patients. Much of my education came from watching my upper-level residents and attending physicians manage these interactions, as well as developing my own techniques. The two sides of this doctor-patient conversation could come together in an unpredictable fashion. As a physician, I faced the dilemma of the optimum approach to communication—barren brutal honesty versus flowery, hopeful depictions? Patients and their families would absorb the bad news with shock, stoicism and tears. Balancing this "end of life equation" between myself and the patients remains a unique clinical challenge. Ultimately, through my knowledge and compassion, I hoped to allow my terminal patients the ability to achieve a semblance of peace through a frightening dying process.

Rick Zimmerman was a new patient to my practice, in his early thirties, and free of any major health problems. He presented for a general physical, and noted some generalized fatigue which seemed to be unusual. His medical examination was unremarkable except for a few swollen lymph nodes on his neck and underarms, but his blood work told a different story; an elevated white blood cell count with too many of a type of white blood cells called lymphocytes. My concern now heightened, I ordered a detailed analysis of his blood smear which confirmed the diagnosis of chronic lymphocytic leukemia (CLL). Many people can live with this type of leukemia for years without any significant treatment intervention. However, he was in his early thirties, which seemed to be surprisingly early for a CLL diagnosis. My nurse called him and arranged for a follow-up visit with me in the office to discuss his current situation.

When I opened the door into the examination room, Rick looked like he had already been silently crying. He was a semi-trailer truck driver, and multiple vibrant tattoos covered both of his forearms. Interestingly, he was clean shaven, soft spoken, moderately slight of build, and did not fit my preconceived visions of a truck driver; perhaps the macho occupation and the conspicuous body ink was a calculated effort by him to project an image of rebellious masculinity. He wore a dark pair of sunglasses that when removed revealed rosy streaked whites of his eyes encompassed by swollen, dark and sunken eyelids. Clearly he had already calculated a worst-case scenario and was trying to anticipate the severity of his medical report.

I initiated the conversation. "Hi Rick, I suppose that you're wondering why I called you in today."

"Yes Doc, I guess you have some bad news to tell me . . ."

I sensed the icy fear that permeated Rick's spirit and all four corners of the room. Leaning in closer to him, I softened my vocal delivery, a hopeful attempt to convey a message of compensatory warmth and understanding. I reviewed his medical history, exam findings, culminating with his fateful abnormal blood count which served as the lynchpin for all of his concomitant physical anomalies. "Well, Rick, it appears that your test results point to a diagnosis of CLL, chronic lymphocytic leukemia. I'm so sorry to have to share this news with you."

In a painful instant, the dam of emotional restraint that Rick had shored up collapsed. His countenance fell meteorically, and he sobbed uncontrollably like one bearing firsthand witness to an unspeakable tragedy.

"Oh God! I knew it was going to be something terrible! Leukemia! It sounds like such a death sentence . . . I can't believe that this is happening to me . . ."

Shit, I'm losing control of the situation. I made a valiant effort to right the patient ship which had horribly run aground. "Now Rick, we don't know what we are are dealing with right now. We don't have all of the clinical infor—"

"My uncle died of leukemia ten years ago! I sure as hell hope that doesn't happen to me . . . I can't believe that I have cancer . . . Holy smokes!"

After momentarily reeling from his emotional outburst, I felt that I had recovered my bearings enough to reenter the game and readdress the situation. "Rick, I can't even comprehend what you're experiencing right now. I wish that I could give you more information about the nature and stage of the leukemia, and prognosis. I am sorry that we can't do that immediately. We need further testing and the help of a hematology-oncology expert. What I can tell you is this—we are going bust our humps to place this leukemia into remission so that you can continue to live the life of your dreams. OK?"

Mr. Zimmerman at last regained some measure of control over his decimated emotional state. The deep sobs slowly retreated to irregular heaves of despair, then shallow sniffles. "Yeah, I guess so, that's all we can do right now. Let's get started." His appearance appeared so incongruous, the tattooed truck driver exterior with a sensitive, almost childlike personality. I thought to myself, *How is this guy going to perform in an all-out cancer fight? Will he be a warrior or a kitten?* but I instantly set those distractions aside. A quick hug and some answers to a few final questions, then Rick was on his way out the door and on to the oncologist's radar screen.

The cancer team obtained a bone marrow biopsy which confirmed Rick's CLL with one additional element of precautionary information listed on the final report, "Chromosomal deletion present which portends an unfavorable prognosis." Alarmed, I called my consulting oncologist Dr. Bennett for advice. Because of his young age and the concerning bone marrow result, the oncologist wanted the treatment to begin immediately, as opposed to observation. Mr. Zimmerman was maintained on a steady course of chemotherapy for several months, which kept things at bay for a while.

However, eighteen months into his cancer battle, Rick's life tapestry began to unravel. He required hospitalization for secondary infections and a neutropenic fever, which are high temperatures with very little or no white blood cells available for immune defense. When the cancer-fighting compounds complete their dirty business, very few healthy germ-fighting cells remain to mount an anti-infective response. I visited him in the hospital and was struck by how different he looked—now bald from the treatments, bloated and pudgy from repetitive courses of prednisone. It was hard to tell whether Rick was winning the cancer battle—it looked like a stalemate at best.

Fortunately, with the help of the cancer team he managed to extricate himself from the depths of his medical complications and return home to his newlywed wife. But with each passing month the hospitalizations became more frequent, the cancer increasingly aggressive, the situation inexorably bleaker. The CLL condition, often inert for years, had horrifically transformed into a serious large B-cell lymphoma, which was much more difficult to eradicate. Soon, Rick's lymphoma had the upper hand, and like a pack of hungry wild dogs, the malicious cells were menacingly circling for one final devastating attack. His mother called me on an unusually warm May morning, notifying me that he was moving to inpatient hospice for his final days. *A thirty-five-year-old newlywed man!* The entire situation seemed so incomprehensible and devoid of fairness.

Sadly, I made the fateful pilgrimage to the hospital to visit Rick for a final time. Arriving in his room, I found him resting quietly, his brother, young wife and a friend keeping a tearful, resigned vigil. I marveled at his undaunted courage and peaceful contentment as the inevitable end of his life approached. He was strikingly pale, emaciated and not overly communicative given his terminal condition, a far cry from the defiant, tattooed trucker from two years ago. His family regaled me with tales of Rick's mischievousness and irascible wit through the years. The stories were simultaneously uplifting about his luminous personality, while amplifying the degree of his life's tragedy. By the next morning, he was gone to the heavens, death's silent scythe shearing through the vital stalk like darkness overtakes the dusk. Rick inspired me with his understated dignity up to his last moments of life, even in the face of insurmountable odds.

He was gaunt, frail, contracted and reserved, but I developed immediate deep admiration for Kyle Thompson. He was formerly a leading cellist in a local symphony orchestra, a virtuoso who could coax eloquent, silky baritone melodies from his mahogany instrument. Unfortunately, the cruel machinations of multiple sclerosis (MS) had smashed his ability to care for himself, let alone pursue his love of music. As a fellow musician, I tried in vain not to tear up during our visits, knowing that progressive spasticity, weakness and incoordination had synergistically combined to deprive him of his talents. His wife was also an accomplished violinist, and was omnipresent with her husband. He noticed my watery, upset eyes at nearly every visit and reassured me that he had made peace with his fate a long time ago.

For the next several years, like a thief in the night, the MS disease process secretly absconded with what was left of Kyle's abilities. He became progressively weaker to the point that speaking, moving and toileting became torture. When the urinary tract infections began recurring at an alarming rate, requiring increasing frequencies and durations of hospitalization with progressive physical decline, Kyle and his family had finally reached the end of his struggle. I connected him with a hospice service who took wonderful care of him through his final days.

When he passed away at the young age of fifty-six, Mr.
Thompson's life epitomized Schubert's *Unfinished Symphony*;
a tremendous talent producing a beautiful work that death
stopped from being completed. I lamented the tragic health
circumstances that irrevocably prevented Mr. Thompson from
creating the beautiful music which brought so much joy for
others. His wife recounted how a few months after Kyle's passing the world famous cellist Yo Yo Ma came to Milwaukee and
paid a personal tribute to Kyle's talents during a special concert.
It was a very moving, loving homage to an incredibly artistic
human being who too briefly brightened the world with his
orchestral prowess.

A month after Kyle's funeral, I received a lovely thank-you
card from his widow. Within the note she enclosed a photograph
with an aerial view of Mount Rainier, the majestic granite sentinel
which overlooks Kyle's native town of Seattle. Its snowcapped
peak and glaciers reflected the last auburn sunset rays in a warm
spectrum of purple, orange and pink. I imagined the reassuring
constancy of that mountain towering over all of the major stages
of Kyle's young life—the first cello purchased by his parents, early
lessons, honor orchestras, gaining admission to music school,
his first big break with a major symphony.

Viewed through a lens of a positive memory recollection,
I ignored all of the turmoil of his terminal stages of his existence. I contemplated him in another, brighter era, engaged in
an intense practice session as a young healthy man, his elegant
arachnoid fingers dancing up and down the strings, producing
the glorious sounds of his magnum opus. Outside his window,
the bustling Puget Sound and white-topped Olympic Mountains

on the western horizon bore witness to his mastery of his first love, an ornate and warm-sounding concerto.

Although their musical choruses have been silenced here on earth, the stoic deaths of Kyle and others have imprinted a melody of inspiration and wonderment upon my heart which I will remember and cherish forever.

CHAPTER 20

BREACH

August had arrived, and it was time to wrap up my summer job and return back to classes. The evenings were already arriving perceptibly earlier, and some nights a faint chill in the air was palpable. This year, however, was both special and poignant: I was set to begin my first year of medical school, returning back to my favorite stomping grounds at the University of Iowa in Iowa City.

The memory of losing my father the previous December hung prominently in my mind and noticeably clouded my enthusiasm and confidence. I was determined to banish the negative energies and thoughts from my mind while simultaneously embracing the positive potential for a special and rewarding medical career. Understanding the mental and physical demands involved with the first year of medical education, I considered deferring my matriculation for a year to get my head straight, earn extra money for school and get my affairs in order. However, I dismissed this notion virtually out of hand because most of my undergraduate classmate friends were moving on to medical school this fall. I would need their warmth, inspiration and emotional support to get through the challenging moments that inevitably loomed ahead. Even more ominously, I harbored a dark fear that if I did not go back to Iowa City for medical school that fall, there was a possibility that I would never return, and the dream that my father and I nurtured about me becoming a doctor would wither and fade.

On a Saturday morning in late August, I tearfully said goodbye to my mom and my sister, and with a loaded-down maroon Chevy Corsica I set off for the brief ninety-minute trek to Iowa City. It was a trip that I had made literally dozens of times growing up and as an undergraduate student. Under a partly sunny sky I repeated the trip with its quaint and small towns along the way that popped up every five to eight miles or so: Sigourney, Webster, South English, Kinross, Wellman, and finally, Kalona and its unique Amish horse-and-buggy enclave. The landscape was filled with the rich rural tableau of scenes that had comforted me countless times on this journey—old cemeteries, tall aromatic fields of corn with the Kelly-green transitioning to russet, cows and horses grazing lazily in the rolling verdant fields, polite Mennonite men and women gathered around a hayrack at a large family gathering. Heavy bountiful ears of corn bent reverently downward, their pockets filled with the rich harvest of a hard year's work. I took some measure of comfort in the stability and predictability of small-town Iowa living. It was difficult not to admire the people who possessed the courage to set up a life for themselves in a corner of the world often without some of the economic and educational advantages of other urban locales.

At the top of a prominent hill, State Highway 1 gracefully turned, a glistening black diamond ribbon winding its way down into the Iowa River valley and ultimately the object of my pilgrimage, Iowa City itself. It had been so good to me for my four years of biomedical engineering education, and I was counting on more triumphs. As I drove past the iconic golden dome of the Old Capitol, the architectural centerpiece of the university campus, I reflected on a myriad of great memories: friendships established, Hawkeye football Saturdays, bar hopping with my roommates, profound life-changing educational experiences.

Coming back to my revered alma mater also filled me with a sense of trepidation. Iowa City and my hometown of Oskaloosa were only seventy-five miles apart, but the distance seemed infinitely larger to me at that time. The seemingly small geographical gulf between these two cities and parts of my existence had grown into a foreboding cultural chasm. I began asking myself some difficult fundamental questions. What kind of personality do I aspire to be going forward? Am I the affable small-town Iowa boy, or a hard-driving medical student with his heart set on academic honors and success? Do I cling to the time-honored, straightforward traditions of my upbringing, or do I enthusiastically press on to capitalize on the new career opportunities which lie ahead of me these next four years?

A few blocks before my new apartment unit was the massive University of Iowa Hospitals and Clinics complex off to the left-hand side of the street. There were attending physicians and their residents actively walking, consulting and conversing with one another outside the buildings. Driving past, I thought of the countless generations of students and physicians who preceded me and would follow me here for their education and training. Many people in this revered incubator of learning would become highly respected clinicians, groundbreaking researchers, academic and medical heroes. I promised myself at that very moment that I wanted to be a hero of medicine, too, and come through for others during the breaches of illness and trauma. The mystery was just how that dream would come to pass over the succeeding years.

In the medical world, emergent situations arise constantly, in a countless array of contexts. The common thread in this scenario is that a patient is in significant, life-threatening distress, and requires quick thinking and immediate intervention. I have dubbed them the "Oh Shit Moments." The key is to minimize fear and panic and instead focus all of my energies onto the critically ill and unstable patient. These stories, while definitely the most terrifying to recall, are also memorable and inspiring.

I was standing at the nurses' station when she impudently burst forth through the waiting room door.

"Doc, you gotta help me!" she cried out desperately. "My chest hurts like a son-of-a-bitch, and I can't breathe!"

In unison, the nurses and I sprung into action and moved her immediately into the closest open patient room. The triage nurse deftly undid her top and undergarments and began placing the leads on for the 12-lead ECG.

"What's your name, ma'am?" I asked.

"Mary . . ."

"When did this pain start?"

"About an hour ago, all of a sudden after I took the garbage to the curb."

"Does it feel like a pressure, like an elephant standing on your chest?"

"Oh God, yes!" She looked ashen, diaphoretic and very uncomfortable.

"Full-strength aspirin, chewed and swallowed now, followed by one sublingual nitro please," I called out to my staff. "Mary, does the pain move anywhere?"

"Yes, all over my chest, shoulder and back!"

"Some of the worst pain that you have ever experienced?"

"Yes, that's for sure!"

"OK, let's get O2 at two liters per minute started for her, and call 911 immediately."

"Already been done!" was the response from the staff.

At this point the ECG had been completed, and the paper tracing spat out on top of the machine. I grabbed the sheet and with an initial perusal my own heart quickly sank: ST segment elevation throughout the graph, consistent with an anterior wall myocardial infarction, or heart attack. I turned my attention back to Mary, now more comfortable as the sublingual nitroglycerin had time to kick into effect.

"OK Mary, it looks like you are having a serious heart attack. We've called 911 and the ambulance will be taking you to the hospital soon."

"Alright, that's what I was afraid was goin' on, anything to make this godawful pain go away."

Almost on cue, the paramedics arrived, and upon taking the report from us, completed their own brief history and assessment, and whisked her off into the ambulance and over to the emergency department, where she would require an emergent cardiac catheterization and angioplasty. I had already given a heads-up to the ER doc and my cardiology colleague, Dr. Jansen. Later in the afternoon, he called me with an update.

"Her left anterior descending (LAD) coronary artery was completely occluded, but I was able to pass a wire through it and ballon angioplasty and stent the blockage down to less than 10 percent. She is doing much better now. Kudos to you and your team, Bruce, your quick thinking and team's performance today saved her life."

"Gee thanks," I humbly uttered in response. "Thanks for keeping me updated, Barry."

As I replaced the receiver, the entire sequence of events seemed surreal to me. It didn't strike me as being dramatic nor heroic in the heat of the battle, simply an emergency which needed to be addressed and we successfully accomplished.

The receptionist came back and knocked on my office door. Her typical sunny countenance was creased with worry and fear on a deceptively calm March morning.

"Dr. Rowe, Mrs. Kostner is here, her son Mason seems quite ill. Is it OK if I send her back here right away for you take a look at her?"

"Sure go ahead, I will be right there."

The waiting room door burst open with tremendous velocity, with such force as if the door was on the verge of flying off of its hinges. Mrs. Kostner came running in, sobbing, holding three-year-old Mason in her arms. He was limp, pale, gasping for air, facial expression enveloped in sheer terror. His respirations sounded obstructive and stridorous, and a perfectly timed seal-like barking cough indicated that most likely this was croup, as opposed to severe pertussis, and no severe drooling to suggest epiglottitis.

"Dr. Rowe, you gotta help us! Mason woke up this morning with a terrible cough and now he can't breathe! I'm so scared!"

In situations like these, stabilizing the patient takes precedence over extended questions and detailed physical examination. I instructed the nurses to call 911 immediately, then checked Mason's oxygen saturation with the pulse oximetry machine. It only read 85 percent, normal is 94 percent and higher as a rule. After an oxygen mask was placed, I gave him a dose of aerosolized racemic epinephrine. The epinephrine shrinks the swelling of the oropharyngeal tissues so that, hopefully, he could temporarily breathe more safely. The treatment helped—he seemed less distressed, with moderately less coughing and stridor, and his pulse oximetry level rose up to 90 percent; not normal, but a definitive improvement. However, in the occasional scary world of croup, we were not out of the woods yet, as the croup episodes can recur hours later with equal severity.

Thankfully, the ambulance arrived in short order and transported Mason to the Children's Hospital for further treatment. Mason made a full recovery; but in the course of the follow-up visits, his mother confided in me that it was one of the worst cases of croup that Children's Hospital had ever seen, requiring a five-day extended hospitalization. Mason never had any further childhood episodes of croup, but I never forgot the fear and terror inscribed on the faces of him and his mother. I felt fortunate to have played a critical role in his initial stabilization and treatment, which allowed the specialists at the tertiary pediatric care hospital to definitively eradicate a life-threatening airway complication.

It was dinnertime on a Saturday, and it had been a busy day for our family. My middle daughter, four-year-old Chelsea, and I had just completed a "Dad and me" swim lesson at the local YMCA. Chelsea hated the class—the water was too cold for her, and she didn't like the games, singing and the swimming activities at all. She was cold, tired and crabby, and now just wanted to eat supper. Our family sat down for a simple dinner, ready to wind down after all of the day's activities.

Abruptly the lightning bolt of terror shattered the atmosphere of irritated boredom. Chelsea took a piece of cantaloupe in her mouth, and emitted what sounded like a gasp followed by faint cough. Startled, I looked up from my plate directly across the table at her, and found her panic-stricken, her eyes wide and searching for salvation. She began to flail her arms wildly and repetitively coughed and searched for aeration—*Dammit, holy shit she's choking!*

My wife spoke first. "Bruce . . ." she said inquisitively and with a palpable increasing level of alarm throughout the course of that monosyllabic sound.

I didn't notice too much, because I had already sprung from my chair and was immediately next to Chelsea. In my panic, I did a finger sweep of her mouth, usually a clinical no-no in the scenario of choking. I could not feel any obvious food material. A moderate back blow between the shoulder blades failed to dislodge the offending obstruction either. I knew that I had a significant choking situation on my hands now, and my daughter's life and future were now at stake. Gruffly I pulled Chelsea from her booster seat and began to perform the lifesaving exercise for all choking victims, the Heimlich Maneuver. With a panicked rapidity I positioned myself behind my second-born, wrapped my arms around her midsection, and after locking my hands and fists together, thrust upward once into her upper abdominal and lower chest cavity. *Nothing.* The choking calamity ominously continued, and a terrifying realization upwelled in my mind. I may have only fifteen brief seconds remaining before she would lose consciousness, and then the crisis would deepen to a new and frightening level. I can't even contemplate the unspeakable horror to follow if I failed my daughter now.

The second and third thrusts were more urgent and with a degree of force that under normal circumstances should never be inflicted upon a child. Leniency had to be abandoned when doing battle with a looming possibility of death. On the third thrust, I pushed upward nearly at full strength, not wanting to harm my little girl but also fully aware of the stakes involved. At the conclusion of that unkind brutal bear hug, an ugly, blood-stained orange piece of the culprit fruit came bursting forth from Chelsea's mouth and landed sickeningly onto the kitchen table.

She regained her ability to breathe unimpeded, and her vio-laceous color returned to normal. Relief and nervous exhaustion washed over the entire horrifying tableau. My wife, Chelsea, and big sister Allison all began uncontrollable crying simultaneously.

Baby Julia was too young to realize the frightening episode which transpired a few feet in front of her. Emotionally spent and exhausted, I slumped back in my chair, appetite completely stolen away from me. While I am thankful that I possessed the strength and the ability to save my young daughter, I also developed a significant fear of the combination of cantaloupe and children.

I was a second-year attending physician, and my partner's patient was in labor at our downtown hospital. Ellen McDonald was admitted for a vaginal birth after cesarean section, or VBAC for short. Her pregnancy had been uncomplicated, and there were no indications that any frightening complications would arise on her delivery. She had presented earlier that morning after her water broke and began contracting with regularity and increasing force. The external monitors were having a difficult time picking up the baby's heart rate and contractions. As a result, I placed an internal heart monitor electrode harmlessly on the baby's scalp and an intrauterine catheter to measure her true contractions. This significantly helped me to accurately monitor her labor pattern. My OB consult, Dr. Farrell, felt comfortable with our current treatment plan.

As the afternoon progressed, Ellen's contractions and cervical dilatation progressed appropriately, but the L&D nurse noticed something unusual—she was having a small of amount of bright red blood vaginally. Often this is a result of "bloody show," which occurs as the cervix magically and exponentially stretches under the pressure and stress of the baby's head. Still, it seemed like a little bit more bleeding than expected in this clinical setting. I erroneously reassured myself that this was a normal variant of VBAC labor and planned to closely monitor her for any further changes and abnormalities in her clinical picture.

At around 4:00 p.m. the bleeding became a bit more pronounced, and then in a flash, the entire labor process spun out of control. The baby's heart tones dramatically decreased, and the pressure catheter ceased to give any readout of data. A definitive catastrophic event had taken place, but what? Something had to be done immediately to deliver this baby. For a couple of seconds I froze.

"Dr. Rowe . . . we gotta do something," the nurse called out.

"Ready for crash section?" asked Dr. Mike Crookham, a third-year OB resident.

"Yes—let's go, let the in-house on call attending know—Mike, you take lead and I'll assist."

With a rapid disconnect of all of the tubes, wires, and sensors, we wheeled Mrs. McDonald into the OR suite, where fortunately the anesthesia attending had already positioned herself for the emergent surgical delivery. With astonishing swiftness we transferred her from her bed to the operating table, and after a brief surgical preparation and rapid induction of general anesthesia, my resident proceeded with the Pfannenstiel incision to free the baby from its terrifying existence. As we dissected the surface layers down to the peritoneum, a sickening discovery—a dark brown-red discoloration was present, indicating a uterine rupture and the extruded placenta lying underneath the translucent surface. After further brief dissection, Dr. Crookham freed the baby from its tenuous intrauterine situation and placed the baby girl on the bassinette.

Fortunately she seemed fine, and the entire process from wheeling out of the labor room to delivery of the infant was a remarkably fast seven minutes. I thanked Dr. Crookham and the team for their support, quick thinking and actions. Then, with a humble and heavy heart, made a quiet and contemplative drive back home that evening. Everyone on the L&D floor seemed so quiet that day. *Were they mad at me? Should I have ordered the C-section sooner, with the increased bleeding, even though by all accounts the baby was stable on the heart rate monitor?*

The next morning, I made rounds on both Mrs. McDonald and her baby girl, Bella. Both had been through a great ordeal yesterday, but surprisingly both seemed to be recovering nicely. The mother was ebullient, thankful, and even managed a weak smile at me.

"Thanks Dr. Rowe, for saving my life and my baby," she expressed reverently. "We were lucky to have you around yesterday."

"You're welcome, Mrs. McDonald, but in reality it was an entire team that recognized the crisis and sprung into action and performed at their best to rescue you and baby Bella."

"I'm so blessed that everything seems to have worked out OK," she replied happily.

"Yes—that's truly the best reward of all." I was grateful for her kind words and appreciation, but remained haunted by the possibility that my performance could have been better and that some long-term complication in the mother or infant was bound to arise.

For many years, I often thought about Mrs. McDonald and baby Bella, and how they were doing, as they were my partner's patients. The answer came to me eighteen years later. As I was standing at the nurses' station, a middle-aged couple approached me from down the hallway. They appeared to be happy, in love, and looked at me with a gratifying kindness.

"Excuse us, are you Dr. Rowe?" they inquired politely.

"Why yes, I am," I responded, my curiosity piqued.

"I'm Ellen MacDonald, and this is my husband Gary. Eighteen years ago you delivered my daughter Bella with an emergent C-section. Just wanted to tell you once again how much we appreciated your quick thinking and quality care that you gave us. Bella will be a freshman at the University of Wisconsin-Madison this fall, studying neuroscience. Thanks again so much!"

"You're so very welcome," I replied, overwhelmed with emotion and trying to maintain my composure. "Those are some of the kindest words anyone has ever said to me during my medical practice. I'm so glad everyone is doing well. You just made my year."

We quickly exchanged hugs, and like many of life's incredible and beautiful moments, it concluded and the drumbeat of reality resumed. I sensed the admiring eyes of my coworkers and fellow docs focused upon me—was I too hard on myself all those years ago? My team and I operated effectively in the critical moments and rescued a mom and baby from potential death and long-term health complications. Everyone else saw the blessed end results, and not the minor blemishes in the process. Knowing that my presence in a crisis medical situation, albeit terrifying, allowed for the betterment of someone else's life was a precious gift. I am grateful for the opportunities afforded to me through family medicine which have equipped me to jump into the breach of life-threatening emergencies and make a positive impact.

CHAPTER 21

LUMINOUS

The concept of light is a powerful, positive concept with far-reaching scientific, social and literary consequences. Albert Einstein grasped the concept of the speed of light, known by the constant letter c, as the ultimate speed limit of the universe in his theories of relativity. In religious settings, Moses interacted with the burning bush in the Old Testament, and Jesus came down from the mountain illuminated as bright as the sun in the Gospel. People who have returned from near-death experiences frequently describe a warm, welcoming bright white light which beckoned them hither. Often in classic literature and film, people such as Ebenezer Scrooge "see the light" and have a change of heart, or like Darth Vader undergo a character rehabilitation and "come back into the light." I have often felt a warm luminous sense of joy with my patients when everything went according to plan, with healthy outcomes and happy patients.

It was early June of '72, and after four years of living and eight tonsillitis episodes, my exasperated parents decided that it was high time that I finally had my tonsils and adenoids removed. For a young child who knew nothing about the mechanics of medicine or hospitals, I was scared as shit. On the fateful surgical day, they put me in a cute little gown and a bouffant cap that made me look like a floret of blue broccoli. Following a short "buggy ride" down the hallway, I found myself in a frightening place. I could only see everyone's eyes; everything else on their bodies was concealed with masks, caps and gowns. A neutral-sounding voice told me to move off of the buggy and onto the table in the center of the room. I nervously did as I was told and laid on my back looking up at the ceiling. The gowned people inexorably closed in around me, compounding my insecurity and claustrophobia.

One person came over by my head and looked down on me. He had an imposing build, and his bulky sausage fingers faintly smelled of tobacco, just like my father's. With a routine clinical bearing, he held a small mesh-like metal basket above my face.

"Take a couple of deep breaths now," he methodically instructed.

The mesh colander thing smelled like a noxious gas, and I fought the urge to panic or run away. *What's happening? Where's Mommy and Daddy? Are these strange people going to hurt me?*

As I began to breathe as I was told, I caught my anesthesiologist's eyes one last time. They projected confidence and comfort, just what a scared young boy needed. A bright overhead light surrounded his countenance like a beautiful halo. His parting words to me were simple but reassuring:

"Relax son, everything's goin' to be alright, we'll take good care of you." Then everything dramatically faded to black until it was all over.

He was correct—everything with the surgery progressed according to plan, and when it was over, I ate an exorbitant amount of ice cream. When my patients are struggling with a serious illness, I fondly remember my anesthesiologist's simple kindness, and bring my light of hope to the darkest corners of their discouragement.

Julia is my youngest daughter and always has charmed me with her friendly nature, positive attitude and a beautiful smile that can quickly illuminate any room. She has also been prone to occasional bouts of unexpected mischief. When my little Juju was only three years old, while on a trip to my in-laws' home in small-town Iowa, she was sitting on Grandma's lap at the dinner table eating some frozen corn. A few minutes later she announced to the table, "I just put a piece of corn in my nose."

"What?" my wife Laura immediately responded. "Which side?"

"This one," she replied matter-of-factly, pointing at her right nostril.

I grabbed a flashlight and directed its beam up the involved nasal passage. Sure enough, a rounded yellow sphere cozily protruded along the inferior turbinate. It was snugly lodged and looked like it may not come out easily.

"We've gotta go the ER tonight," I concluded. "The kernel of corn is organic material, it could swell overnight and be even more of a problem tomorrow."

Laura's hometown of Mount Pleasant, Iowa, was similar in size and feel to my native Oskaloosa. As a result, I called the emergency department in town, identified myself as a licensed

Wisconsin physician, and requested to bring my daughter in for an evaluation. I took the unusual step of asking for equipment to be set aside for a foreign body removal—MacGill forceps, anesthetic spray and some gauze. The ER receptionist was not unnerved by this comment. "OK," she replied nonchalantly, "we'll have it ready for you."

Twenty minutes later Laura, Juju and I arrived at the ER, simply identifying myself as the doctor who called in advance about the child with the foreign body. Without asking for any identification or registration, a friendly nurse escorted us back to a small patient room where all of the equipment that I had requested was neatly set into place. Wasting no time on this pleasantly warm April evening, I set to work. I gently laid Julia down on the gurney and adjusted the overhead light toward her nose to get good visualization of the mischievously hiding corn kernel.

"Juju, I am going to put some spray into your nose so that it won't hurt when I take the piece of corn out of your nose, OK sweetie?"

"OK Daddy, I'll be good."

I coated the nasal mucosa with a gentle jet of topical anesthetic, which Julia tolerated well. However, when I turned to grab the forceps, Juju took matters into her own hands. With a dramatic arch of her back, followed by a brisk recoil and lurching forward, she made an unmistakeable sound:

"AAAHCHOO!"

In a dramatic instant, the entrapped nugget of corn ejected itself and landed squarely on the teddy bear woven on the front of Julia's pajamas. I double-checked her nostril for any other retained pieces of corn; finding none, we were clearly finished.

The entire process took less than ten minutes and without any of the paperwork and bureaucracy that is inherent in typical medical encounters. I marveled at the level of trust and comfort that the small-town hospital placed in an unknown out-of-town doctor.

Three weeks into my career as an attending physician, standing at my nurses' station, I noticed my one o'clock patient gingerly walk in, hunched over and tentative in his overall bearing. Patrick McCurdy was forty-eight years old and had noticed some abdominal pain for the last twenty-four hours. Entering the patient room I attempted to identify the nonverbal cues that a patient is exhibiting. Patrick looked hunched over and uncomfortable.

"Hi Mr. McCurdy, I am Dr. Rowe, one of the new physicians here at the Glendale Clinic. You look like you are not feeling so hot right now."

"Yes Doc, that is an understatement . . . my stomach is killing me."

"When did it start?"

"I'm not sure, maybe yesterday morning?"

"Is it getting better, worse or staying about the same?"

"Clearly getting worse, it hurts pretty bad, Doc."

On examination Patrick had a significantly tender abdomen, in a diffuse region over the middle right side. He had tightness of his abdominal musculature both before and after pushing down on his belly with my examining hands, conditions referred to as voluntary and involuntary guarding. Guarding can indicate significant intra-abdominal inflammation and infection. The location of pain was not in the classical right lower quadrant area of acute appendicitis, nor in the right upper quadrant region seen with an inflamed gallbladder, called cholecystitis.

Momentarily I was somewhat stumped, but then a lightbulb went off in my head. Occasionally the tail of an infected swollen appendix can hide behind the back of the colon, a condition referred to as retrocecal appendicitis. Mr. McCurdy's presentation appeared to be consistent with this medical condition. Further enhancing my suspicion was an elevated white blood cell count with an increase in the fraction of immature white cells. I reviewed my findings with Patrick and enlisted the consultative services of a general surgeon, Dr. Oscarson. A followup CT scan confirmed the appendicitis diagnosis, and he underwent surgery later that afternoon. As I was finishing up my afternoon clinic, the hot line phone jangled to life. It was Dr. Oscarson.

"Hey Bruce, Jack here. You were right on the money. A retrocecal appendicitis. You caught it early and no perforation occurred. His surgery went well, and I don't anticipate any long-term complications. Nice job!"

"Thanks Jack, much appreciated." I replaced the receiver and brightly walked down my office hallway, ebullient and buoyant in each successive stride.

As I turned to walk out of the exam room, Greg sprung the dreaded "hand on the doorknob question." These last-minute inquiries can range from innocently benign, such a checking out a mole, to a potentially life-threatening piece of information like severe depression. Greg's voluntary disclosure was nonspecific but had a wide range of potential clinical implications.

"So Doc, I have been having this chest pain recently . . ."

Greg was in his mid-forties, somewhat overweight and had a family history of coronary artery disease, which raised my concern about his symptoms. A baseline ECG in the office that day looked normal, but that was not sufficient to be reassuring. He was going to require a stress test for a more in-depth evaluation, consisting of walking on a treadmill of increasing speed and incline with ECG and symptom monitoring for around ten minutes.

Two days later, Greg returned to our office for his formal cardiac testing. He was young and appeared relatively healthy, so I was not anticipating any significant drama that morning. However, only about three minutes into his walking, clearly something was already amiss. The ST segment on the ECG tracing, normally a level flat line after the QRS spike everyone sees on TV medical dramas, began to rise precipitously. Changes on the ST segment during the exercise stages of stress testing are ominous and can indicate serious problems with the blood flow to various areas of the heart. About five minutes into the test his ST line was about 3 mm higher than the level present at the baseline, a huge difference. I was stunned at what I was witnessing: This situation indicated that Greg had significant coronary disease and was at imminent risk for a heart attack.

Based upon superficial physical appearances, I never would have expected this outcome just a few short minutes ago. As I was digesting this profoundly troubling piece of clinical information, two more further problematic findings crystallized to confirm my strong suspicions about Greg's serious heart disease diagnosis. The first was a comment from the patient himself:

"OK Doc, here comes that chest pain again that I felt last week."

"Did it start just now?" I replied with escalating concern and nervousness.

""Uh . . . about a minute ago, pressure right in the middle of my chest, getting worse now."

Right after he completed that sentence, a secondary alarming finding occurred on the ECG. Greg had a five-beat run of a serious, life-threatening arrhythmia called ventricular tachycardia (VT). I was appropriately terrified and had seen enough worrisome findings on the stress test for one day. Immediately his test was terminated, and over a few minutes his ECG returned to normal, deceptively as if nothing had ever happened. A nitroglycerin tablet placed under his tongue relieved the sinister, lurking anterior chest wall pain at least for the time being.

Greg was sent to the hospital, and the following day a cardiac catheterization confirmed the diagnosis: a 99 percent blockage of the primary coronary artery over the front of the heart called the left anterior descending artery (LAD). After an angioplasty and stent placement, the narrowing was completely mitigated and, Greg continued to live a full life symptom- and incident-free. I felt honored to identify a life-threatening medical illness in Greg so that his light of life could continue to burn for many more years.

All of the third-year residents in my program were required to complete a one-month stint in the neonatal intensive care unit (NICU) in our training hospital. I loved caring for and learning from the newborn babies of a variety of weights, sizes and medical conditions. Some of the infants were quite seriously ill, and I took comfort that the unit was staffed with 24-hour neonatologist coverage that was only a phone call away.

On an early spring evening, Jacob was transferred over from labor and delivery for further observation. He was born approximately five weeks before his due date, which often does not present significant issues. The pregnancy, labor and delivery history was uncomplicated, with the exception of his early arrival. Jacob's assessment was unremarkable, except for some increased congestion on his lung examination. A chest X-ray showed some prominent markings in his lungs, which may have been consistent with some retained fluid in the chest, a so-called "wet lung." His respiratory rate was a little bit higher than normal, which often manifests in neonates as transient tachypnea of the newborn. Over the next few hours, however, Jacob's breathing was not improving as expected. His breathing rate remained rapid, had continued coarse breath sounds and, more ominously, exhibited the grunting, nasal flaring and exaggerated muscle action below the bottom of his rib cage referred to as subcostal retractions. These were the subtle but clearly noticeable signs of an infant in worsening respiratory distress.

Attempting to extricate myself from my deepening sense of concern and unease, I paged my neonatology attending. "Hello, Dr. Fuller? It's Bruce Rowe, senior resident on the NICU at Waukesha Memorial Hospital. I have a thirty-five-weeker here that isn't breathing so hot. I think he may have RDS [respiratory distress syndrome]. He may need surfactant. Can you please come and give me a hand?"

"Absolutely Bruce, will be right there," Dr. Fuller crisply replied.

About twenty-five minutes later, Dr. Fuller arrived and completed his assessment on the baby. His diagnosis and the appraisal of the situation were congruent with mine. He instructed the nurse to get the equipment ready to deliver surfactant to the baby.

"What kind of gloves do you need?" the nurse requested kindly.

"Ask Bruce—he has been diligently watching his patient all night, he's going to be delivering the surfactant treatment."

Surfactant is a compound delivered to premature babies to help them breathe more efficiently. In normal-term infants, the lung tissue naturally inflates after delivery like a graceful, gossamer balloon. In premature infants, however, the surface tension on the lung tissue remains very high, and it is difficult to get the lungs expanded. I liken it to the Herculean effort that it takes to blow up one of those long, tight circus animal-type balloons. The surfactant medication, a soapy-like substance, reduces the surface tension in the microscopic alveoli of the lung tissues, allowing for them to expand and function normally. It had only come onto the market just a few months before that time, and I was anxious to see if would be effective in Jacob's case.

"Bruce, I am going to talk you through this. I'll be right beside you here but I want you to do this case, alright?"

"Sure, Dr. Fuller," I responded with nervous excitement. "I think we're about ready."

I placed a temporary endotracheal tube in Jacob's airway and with a small ambubag gently administered a few puffs of supplemental oxygen. Subsequently, with more rapid small squeezes of the bag I aerosolized the lifesaving surfactant into my vulnerable baby's lungs. A few moments later, we were finished—the breathing tube was removed and he was placed back under an oxygen hood. Now all that I could do was simply wait and see whether our efforts were ultimately successful.

It didn't take long. Over the next ninety minutes, Jacob's respiratory rate, oxygenation levels and breathing struggles all improved dramatically. Another thirty minutes elapsed, and it was clear that the immediate pulmonary crisis was over. The speed and magnitude of the respiratory turnaround in this beautiful, young life on the infant warmer in front of me was completely stunning. Almost on cue, I felt a warm, pleasant arm gracefully drape around my shoulder in a professional sideways embrace. It was Dr. Fuller.

"Nice job, Bruce . . . you saved his life! Pretty good feeling, huh?"

"Yeah, that's an understatement," I replied, feeling a mixture of pride and being overwhelmed. "I just didn't think that he would turn around that quickly."

"Pretty amazing stuff, that surfactant. Prior to this we had a lot of difficult and tragic cases. See you tomorrow for rounds, Bruce." In an instant, he disappeared into the night.

"OK, sounds good." I gazed out the large airy windows of the unit, designed to let in as much light as possible. So many hours had passed without my knowledge that evening had yielded to dusk, only to be overtaken by the velvet darkness. My heart inside was as bright as midday, thrilled that my baby was recovering and that I played a pivotal role.

As I drove home that evening, I also reflected on my lessons of history, and that this case was similar to that of one Patrick Bouvier Kennedy, son of John F. Kennedy and Jacqueline Kennedy, with one tragic exception. Born a few weeks early in 1963, Patrick did not have the benefit of surfactant medication and died shortly after birth. The fact that in this era he would have not only survived, but gone on to live a long, healthy life served as a poignant counterpoint to my successful newborn case that night.

In the beige-colored environs of the Children's Hospital Emergency Room, my sick baby made a gloomy and unceremonious entrance. Brett was only three weeks old, but had a fever of 101.8 degrees Fahrenheit. Fever in young infants is not a good diagnostic sign, and in children less than two to three months of age requires an aggressive evaluation and workup. His initial physical examination was normal, but he would need to be admitted, started on IV antibiotics and have cultures obtained. Usually this would require blood, urine and cerebrospinal fluid cultures, the latter obtained from a lumbar puncture (LP), also known as a spinal tap. As the lead resident on Brett's case, I was scheduled to perform the LP, which I had performed a few times previously with varying success.

Dr. Katie Patton was my attending ER physician that evening. I respected her no-nonsense approach to pediatric emergency medicine and her high expectations of excellence from her residents. "OK Bruce, if you get a champagne tap on this baby, I'm bringing you in a bottle of wine."

A champagne tap refers to an LP performed with such technical skill that no red blood cells contaminate the sample. Usually in most cases a couple of red blood cells meander into the collection tube, and while not enough to contaminate or obscure the test results, is sufficient to disqualify the LP procedure as perfect.

After discussing the situation with Brett's anxious parents and obtaining their informed consent, I set up my procedure tray and got Brett prepared for the spinal tap. I located the two successive midline back bumps called spinous processes at around the L4-L5 levels and copiously cleaned the area with Betadine. My nurse with compassionate firmness placed Brett into a forced C-shaped fetal position, his convex lumbar spine protruding curiously out toward me, brilliantly illuminated by the targeted surgical light positioned above us.

I placed the spinal needle between the two spinous process, angling slightly upward toward his head. I heard a slight gasp from Brett, followed by a shocked and deep-seated astonished crying. While saddening and unsettling, I needed to temporarily ignore his discomfort in the name of medical diagnosis and treatment. I removed the sheath insert from the spinal needle, gave it a ninety degree turn and . . . success! Immediately the healthy-appearing, clear cerebrospinal fluid steadily exuded in small rivulets. The transparent fluid color was a reassuring clinical sign. I collected three small tubes for protein, glucose, cell counts and culture, sent them off, removed the needle and placed a small Band-Aid over the puncture mark. Brett's sobs had subsided into a quiet sad resignation and relief that the episode of discomfort had elapsed.

The quiet reverent silence was broken by Dr. Patton. I didn't realize that she had been quietly watching me from behind. "Way to go, Bruce! This could be a champagne tap for you."

"Thanks Dr. Patton, as long is Brett is OK, that's all the reward that I will need."

All of the news going forward for my patient Brett was great. He was hospitalized for forty-eight hours on IV antibiotics with ampicillin and gentamicin, his cultures were are all negative, and he made a full recovery from what appeared to be a short-lived but alarming viral infection. The spinal fluid sample viewed under the microscope showed nary a red blood cell! *My first champagne tap!*

At the conclusion of my next shift, a bottle of Cabernet Sauvignon awaited me, with a small note included:

Dear Dr. Rowe,

Great LP technique, excellent patient care, and a "champagne" spinal tap performed with no red blood cells. This bottle of wine is for you. Strong work!

Yours,
Dr. Patton

It is always gratifying when you perform your job well and receive positive acknowledgement for your accomplishments from your superiors. To this day, I try to follow Dr. Patton's example and build up the confidence in my fellow health-care team members by shining my light of support upon them, through education, creating a teamwork atmosphere in medical decision-making, or simple encouragement.

Elaine was a thirty-year-old single mother of two that I had known for just a couple of years. Most of her issues revolved around the anxiety and stress of being the sole parent of two young children. On a stormy summer day she came into the office noticeably more concerned and stressed than her normal baseline.

"Dr. Rowe, I think something is really wrong with my right eye. It is really blurry and I can't see much out of it, just dark spots and bright lights."

"Did this come on all of a sudden?"

"Yes it did."

"Any headaches, other neurologic symptoms such as weakness, numbness, tingling, difficulty speaking, or the like?"

"Nope—just this weird eye thing."

"Any history of eye problems previously?"

"None except for needing glasses for nearsightedness."

Elaine's initial assessment, including a full neurological check, was completely normal. When I flashed the light into her right eye, however, things seemed very strange indeed. In an ophthalmoscopic examination it is important to examine the rear of the eye chamber and locate a silvery or yellowish circle called the optic disc. This disc represents the entry point of the optic nerve and the blood vessels into the back of the eye called the retina. Abnormalities of the disc can be a harbinger of a variety of ophthalmic and neurologic issues including glaucoma and brain tumors. When I attempted to examine Elaine's optic disc in the right eye, I was befuddled. *I cannot find the disc at all!* After several efforts and my patient becoming increasingly light sensitive, I abandoned my attempts to complete the examination. Increasingly alarmed, I contacted Ted Lewis, one of the nearby ophthalmologists to convey my findings and request a stat referral.

"Are you sure, Bruce, that you couldn't find the disc?"

"Yes Dr. Lewis, it was plain as day in the left eye, but for the life of me I can't identify it in the right eye. I'm pretty good with the ophthalmoscope."

"OK, send her over later this morning, I guess," he replied noncommittally. He appeared to be unmoved by my assessment, and I was annoyed that my specialist's concern for Elaine was not congruent with mine.

An hour later, my vindication arrived through an urgent phone call from the ophthalmologist's office. Dr. Lewis wanted to speak with me immediately. The voice on the other end of the line was animated with a hint of contriteness.

"Holy crap, Bruce! This lady has optic neuritis, and that is why you could not find the optic disc in her right eye. I am going to obtain some blood work and refer her to a neurologist and for an urgent MRI to rule out multiple sclerosis. Does that sound reasonable?"

Unbelievable, I was right. I stood by the phone, stunned at the turn of events, paralyzed momentarily about how to respond. Not only was my poor-man's eye examination correct, it indicated a serious medical diagnosis. "Sure, that sounds good, Dr. Lewis. I appreciate the update and thanks for seeing her so quickly."

"You're welcome, Bruce, any time." The call quickly terminated.

Elaine was referred for follow-up tests and consultation, but unfortunately she moved to Minneapolis and was lost to follow-up. I think of her often and hope that her vision recovered and no other worrisome diagnoses were uncovered. A small light in my hand and a basic examination of the eye proved to be the brilliantly illuminating window into Elaine's diagnosis.

It was an unseasonably cool summer Saturday evening, and my wife and I were driving home from a relaxing, enjoyable dinner at one of our favorite Japanese restaurants.

"The bento box was really good tonight, don't you think?" I asked.

"Yes, not bad," Laura replied, fulfilled and sleepy. "I thought that the yellowfin tuna was even more outstanding than usual."

Before I had a moment to register my agreement, my pager inconveniently jangled to life, rudely interrupting our joyful couple's reverie. At a stop light I glanced down at the number in the display. It was the number that had appeared on my screen on a multitude of occasions, the emergency department. I punched the number into my cell phone and was connected to one of my favorite emergency department docs, Kevin O'Brien, an excellent diagnostician who had a wonderful manner with people. He quickly picked up my return phone call.

"Hey Bruce, it's Kevin, how goes it tonight?" he quipped, displaying a positive energy that could erode as a challenging evening shift wore on.

"Hi Kev, goin' well here, what's up?"

"Well, I got this nice eighty-two-year-old gentleman patient of Dr. Stephenson's, his name is Joseph Pardubsky, having a lot of coffee-ground emesis and black tarry stools, looks like an upper GI bleed. Currently he is hemodynamically stable, but his red count is down and he takes some potent blood thinners. I got him typed and crossed for four units of blood, and I think we need to put him in the unit at least for observation. Sound good?"

"Yes—agree totally with that plan," I politely assented, somewhat disappointed that my call weekend would now be wrapped up with a potentially medically challenging and unstable patient. I called in orders and planned to see him very early the next morning unless his condition suddenly deteriorated.

At around 5:00 a.m. the pager, now at my bedside, impolitely squawked again. This time it was the ICU calling, and Carrie, one of the top nurses in our hospital, was on the other end of the line.

"Dr. Rowe, Mr. Pardubsky isn't looking too good right now. His systolic blood pressure is around 100, and heart rate up to 120 beats per minute, and his hemoglobin dropped from 10 to 8 in the last six hours. The NG tube is draining coffee-ground and bloody-looking fluid. I am uncomfortable with this situation." I always respect the nurses and teammates who have the courage to speak up when they are concerned about a sick patient. In the airline world, it is called Crew Resource Management, where every team member has an equal voice in the flight operation. Whether it is an aircraft or a patient, it is a powerful tool to ensure quality and safety.

"OK Carrie, I will be there in about fifteen to twenty minutes," I replied a little more groggily than I would like. Quickly I got up, threw on a pair of khakis and a basic button-down oxford, tieless, and made my way downstairs to my car. These were the mornings where I sometimes wished I became an engineer, and I could read the morning paper and relax with a cup of coffee. The drive to the hospital is normally exactly ten minutes, but being early on a Sunday morning and with my sense of urgency I arrived in about seven. I briskly walked into the ICU wing, attempting to warm up my stethoscope from the cool night air.

"Good morning Carrie," I chirped, now finally beginning to wake up a little bit with the cool morning air and a warm cup of coffee. "What's up with Mr. Pardubsky?"

"No change since I spoke with you a little while ago, he just doesn't look right to me."

Often in medicine, especially with experience, we rely on our gut instincts, and how a patient looks in appearance carries a great deal of weight. A person can have pretty good lab results and X-rays, but if they look significantly ill, it may call for a second look and additional monitoring. Quietly, I entered Mr. Pardubsky's room for an initial assessment. He looked gaunt, haggard and pale, like he had not slept in days.

"Hi there, I'm Dr. Rowe, sounds like you've had a rough couple of days."

"Name's Joe," he replied with a prominent aura of tiredness and worry. "What's goin' on, Doc? I feel like crap and completely wiped out."

"You have anemia, which is a low red blood cell count. Red blood cells carry oxygen, which is critical for survival. Currently your red cell volume, or hemoglobin, is about 50 percent of where it should be. I think that you are bleeding internally from a stomach ulcer, and the blood loss is ongoing."

"What are we going to do about it?" he countered politely.

"Well, we are going to need to give you some blood, probably at least four units, and I will call the GI doctor to take a look in your stomach later this morning. Once we get the bleeding stopped and your red blood cells back to a normal level, we should be back in business."

"I hope so, I've had a lot health problems recently. Just got a stent a couple of months ago, now I am on two blood thinners."

"Yes I know, those are important meds for sure." I had reviewed and stopped his anticoagulation meds last night pending our evaluation today. In the cardiac world aspirin and highly potent additional blood thinners have been utilized with great success. However, for patients like Joe, the now-watery arterial liquid can bleed in quick, unpredictable and terrifying ways. Back at the nurses' station, I updated my stalwart GI doc, Dr. Ellerbee, and prepped Joe for four units of blood. Little did I know that I was entering a twelve-hour pitched battle with death for Mr. Pardubsky's life that would be memorable for both of us.

Noon on Sunday arrived all-too quickly, and things seemed a little bit better with my patient's situation. Mr. Pardubsky had an upper endoscopy completed by the GI team, and a tear in the gastroesophageal junction region had apparently been successfully cauterized. He was on his fourth unit of blood, and his blood counts and vital signs finally appeared to be stabilizing. His wife Mary Ann and her identical twin sister Robin sat side by side on the family couch in the patient's room.

"Tell me, Doctor," Mary Ann said tentatively, "is my Joseph goin' to make it through OK?"

"I'm planning on it," I responded, surprised at my verbal and nonverbal display of confidence. I hoped that it came off as reassuring and comforting, not arrogant. "We certainly are not out of the woods yet, but the outlook is a great deal better than it was earlier this morning."

"Oh thank you, Doctor," she gratefully answered. "I am ever so appreciative of you and the nurses."

"I know you are, and it's our pleasure," I warmly replied. "I'll stay around a little while longer and make sure everything is stable."

Joe's nurse Carrie was now off shift, and fortunately another ace nurse Nicole had taken her place. We reviewed the case and the day's events together.

"Bruce, he seems a little better, but his red blood cell counts have not risen as much as I would like. Plus his blood pressure is hovering around 100 systolic."

"I agree, Nicole, let's give him another two units of blood and have some dopamine on hand in case his blood pressure drops further." dopamine and other drugs like it are called pressor agents, used in the ICU to support a person's blood pressure when their internal organ systems are disabled. I consulted my critical care specialist, Dr. Salmone, who agreed with our plan and would see him later in the afternoon.

Sunday afternoon was peppered with a steady stream of calls from Nicole about Mr. Pardubsky. His blood pressure was labile—sometimes running high, and other times somewhat low. The blood count was dropping again—four more units, now he had received ten units total, a substantial amount for a non-trauma patient. Later in the afternoon, his blood pressure tanked, 100 . . . 90 . . . 80 . . . 75 . . . finally, Nicole had had enough. An early evening phone call to me sounded strained and even alarming.

"Dr. Rowe, I have him on three different pressor drugs, his blood transfusion and IV fluids are running wide open, and I am still having trouble maintaining his blood pressure. I need you here now!"

"On my way," I quickly replied and grabbed my jacket. We had some friends over for a cookout, and upon excusing myself I could sense my wife's frustration at my being mentally and emotionally invested in this case all day. "I'll be back as soon as possible," I lamely reassured her, not knowing what that meant in terms of a timeline.

Arriving back on the floor, I encountered a tableau of frantic medical intervention bordering on pandemonium. Nurses and respiratory therapists hurriedly rushed about, procuring medications and necessary medical supplies for Mr. Pardubsky. I found Nicole hanging a fresh pressor bag at my patient's bedside, reasonable urgency bordering on panic. "Doc, he's not doing well here, what are we going to do?"

At this moment I mentally sensed a tunnel of light enveloping me and focusing exclusively on my patient. All of the initial fear and dark uncertainty seemed to fall away as my thoughts appeared to illuminate and clarify the complicated medical situation in front of me. Strangely, I felt confident in my clinical acumen, immediately knowing what the next steps were going to be in managing my patient. All of the years of my training and experience were converging at this precise, wondrously epochal moment. Athletes often describe this as being "in the zone," where they focus on the task at hand at the exclusion of all other distracting elements. Concentrating on my critically ill patient, the surrounding increasingly anxious and concerned voices receded in my mind while I carefully crafted our next move.

"Max the pressors . . . now!" I commanded. "Dr. Ellerbee will be here momentarily and we will need to re-scope him immediately and locate that stomach bleeder . . . it must still be active. I need four more units of blood up here stat!" I was surprised at the level of volume and directness of my replies.

"Hey Doc, what about—"

"No, that's it for now . . . I need the GI nurses up here ASAP to get ready for this procedure!"

Almost on cue, the GI team and Dr. Ellerbee arrived simultaneously on the unit. Quickly Joe was prepped, sedated, and the scope was passed effortlessly into his esophagus and stomach region. Once in the gastric residence, within the violaceous bloody walls, a steady and slow hemorrhaging stomach ulcer and tear made its presence known. I stared at the oozing crevice in anger, wanting it destroyed with all of my being. Dr. Ellerbee placed three clips over the bleeding sites, and the wondrously unthinkable happened: Joe's bleeding abruptly stopped and his blood pressure stabilized. I thanked the GI team, gave two more units of blood, and spent a couple more hours monitoring him and gradually reducing his fluids and blood pressure-supporting medication.

The next few days were glorious, almost a victory lap of sorts. Joe steadily improved, his bleeding clearly stopped, and red blood counts increased positively with each passing day. The pressors were removed, IV fluids reduced, then discontinued completely. His strength and energy level recovered, and after about a week he was able to go to a rehabilitation unit for a couple of weeks before uneventfully being discharged to home.

A few weeks later, a personal letter addressed to me arrived at the clinic. It was from Joe's wife Mary Ann. Curiously, I opened it, interested in its contents. It read:

Dear Dr. Rowe,

I just don't know how I can write a letter to a doctor to express my gratitude to him for saving my husband's life. So I will just simply say it: Thank you for saving my husband's life. I am eternally grateful for all that you have done for Joe and my family.

Fondly,
Mary Ann Pardubsky

Amazed at the beautiful, simple layout of her prose, I humbly sunk down into my office chair. *Wow, what a heartfelt letter. I can't believe that my role as a doctor could have that type of impact on another human being and their family.*

As the years progressively tick by, it is easy to get caught up in the frustrating day-to-day difficulties of modern medicine. All of the challenges can conspire to create an environment of burnout for a physician. When those moments inevitably arrive, I always think about patients like Mr. Pardubsky and others when I performed at my best as a luminous force of healing, while graciously receiving the reflected light of appreciation from a thankful patient.

CHAPTER 22

HARVEST

Ever since my father passed away, the first week in December has been a difficult time for me. Even though the happy anticipation of Christmas is well underway, the sadness of the anniversary of my father's death often looms large in my mind. A couple of years ago, between some frustrating patient interactions and my depressed spirits, it was shaping up to be a difficult commemoration.

One night, with a snowstorm raging outside, I needed to channel my negative energies into a workout. I bundled up, put on my snowshoes and embarked on a brisk hike through the golf course which abuts my subdivision. The air was cold but not frigid, with a conspicuous absence of wind. Large conglomerations of snowflakes gently fell to the ground, adorning my face and shoulders. As I churned through a spirited lap around the tenth hole, I reflected upon my favorite holiday movie *It's a Wonderful Life*. I recalled protagonist George Bailey struggling to see whether his life and work had purpose and positive impacts on others. When George jubilantly runs through the center of town in a blinding snowstorm after finally realizing the true powerful benefit of his existence, it is a beautiful moment. As the days in a busy medical practice relentlessly fly by, it is tempting to view the process as pure work and not a higher-level vocation. Fortunately, my patients and health-care team have regularly reminded me of the pure joys and rewards of being a family doctor.

Emily Nguyen was a petite, energetic Vietnamese lady who was anxiously anticipating the arrival of her first child. As a young attending physician, I had the privilege of managing her obstetrical care. Her pregnancy had progressed normally without incident well into the third trimester.

About a month before her due date, her uterine measurements began to increase more rapidly than expected. Concerned, I referred her to a high-risk OB specialist called a perinatologist. Fortunately, the baby looked great on the ultrasound exam, with one catch—this looked like it would be a good-sized baby. While generally good news on the surface, it could present a distinct risk in a tiny 5'1" woman for a problem called shoulder dystocia, where the infant gets stuck in the birth canal and becomes a difficult, occasionally terrifying delivery. At that point I realized that we would need to induce her for a delivery prior to her due date. Two weeks before her predicted delivery date, a follow-up ultrasound estimated the baby's weight at ten and a half pounds.

The time had arrived to get Emily's baby into the outside world. After confirming this approach with my OB attending, I brought Emily into the hospital in the evening for an induction of labor, giving her an IV medication called Pitocin to stimulate the uterine contractions.

Overnight, her labor progressed according to plan, with good fetal heart tones on the monitor, strong uterine contractions and a progressively dilating cervix. By 10:00 a.m. she was completely dilated and was determined to push. After an hour of pushing, the baby's head arrived at the birth canal and was ready to be delivered.

"OK Emily—let's give it all you got now!" I called out with half encouragement, half varsity football coach tone in my voice.

"Alrighty, here goes . . ." she meekly replied.

The head expressed itself relatively easily, but was sucked back toward Emily's bottom. My heart sank. *Shit—it's a shoulder dystocia.* The shoulders were tightly wedged up against the pubic bones; there was no way the baby would deliver in this configuration. In my mind I ran through the protocols for treating shoulder dystocia, attempting to remain clear-headed and calm.

"Hey guys—" I called out to no one in particular, "we got dystocia, I need a McRoberts maneuver here."

The McRoberts maneuver consists of bringing the mother's knees up toward her chest in hopes of widening the birth canal geometry for delivery. My nurses quickly complied as I asked. *Nothing.* The baby remained stuck.

"Alright that didn't work, I need some suprapubic pressure please . . ." One of the nurses made a tight fist and pushed down hard on the abdomen right above the pubic bone, hoping to free up the front shoulder. *No progress . . . Oh boy.* I struggled to maintain my sense of composure and not to convey panic. Time for the next plan of attack, the Wood Screw maneuver.

The Wood Screw technique involves the delivering doctor placing their fingertips over both the front and rear shoulders, gently rotating the baby up to 180 degrees in a screw-like fashion.

If it worked, both shoulders should free themselves with successful delivery of the baby shortly thereafter. I prayed that this intervention would succeed, otherwise the crisis would progress to a new, darker level. With some effort, I was able to get the baby rotated, ultimately with some loosening of the shoulders. *Thank God.* It was sufficient enough to free up the baby for delivery.

I brought forth the rest of the baby as slowly and controlled as possible, being careful not to place too much traction on the head and neck. Excessive pulling of this area could traumatize a nerve bundle in the neck area called the brachial plexus and cause arm weakness called an Erb's palsy. If severe enough of an injury, the child could have long-term problems with arm strength and functionality. Gingerly, I coaxed the reluctant infant out of its reclusive habitat. *Man, this kid is huge!* Finally our baby was free and clear of the birth canal hazards, escaped into the outside world. A boy named Andy, exactly ten and a half pounds as predicted. For a few short hours he had some trace arm weakness suspicious of a very mild Erb's palsy; by the next day it had completely resolved without any long-term complications.

A few months ago Andy came into the office for his high school senior year sports physical. He was still imposing, at 6'2" tall, lean, muscular and athletic, planning to play Division III college football as a free safety. I admired his level of fitness and self-confidence, his excitement and optimism for the future. Reflecting back on that momentous day eighteen years ago, I felt blessed to have played a small part in helping Andy arrive into this world healthy and safe.

Jeff Maxwell was forty-two years old, a new patient who came into my office on a sultry July afternoon with a common medical problem: bright red rectal bleeding. With his younger age, frequently the cause is benign internal and external hemorrhoids, as opposed to more sinister pathology. I made a point to take a thorough history with Jeff.

"So Jeff, you've been having some bright red rectal bleeding the last few months?"

"Yep."

"Is it every day, or does it come and go?"

"Seems like it comes and goes a lot."

"Does it stain the toilet tissue, toilet water or mix in with the stool?"

"I would say yes to all of those."

"Any weight loss, extreme fatigue, night sweats or belly pain?"

"Not that I can recall . . ."

"Has there been a lot of bleeding when it occurs?"

"Yes—sometimes it seems like a lot."

"Is it always a bright red bleeding, no black or maroon-colored stools, Jeff?"

"I think so, but I've gotta admit I don't always check very closely."

My exam of Jeff didn't reveal much of significance. There was no abdominal pain, mass or swelling to suggest a colonic tumor. His rectal exam showed a small amount of reddish-brown stool which tested positive for blood. I used an anoscope to look into his anus and rectal area, an awkward undertaking for both doctor and patient, especially the latter. The scope examination showed a few small internal and external hemorrhoids, but nothing actively bleeding.

Something doesn't seem right here. Given the amount of bleeding that he was describing, I would have expected to find larger hemorrhoids, with some evidence of recent blood loss. I was not comfortable chalking this up to simple hemorrhoidal bleeding. Something in my clinical subconscious was nagging at me, convincing me that more testing needed to be done.

"Jeff, I see a few small hemorrhoids down here, but it may not account for all of your bleeding. I think you need to have a colonoscopy performed for a complete evaluation."

He seemed cautious at the prospect. "Are ya sure, Doc? After all, I'm only in my early forties, and there's no history of colon cancer in my family."

"Yes Jeff, I believe this is important. There may be another source of your rectal bleeding besides hemorrhoids, and a colonoscopy would help us a lot."

"OK Doc, if you're concerned about it, then so am I, I'll do the colonoscopy." He was generally polite about the prospect of sedation, a missed day of work and a nearly two-meter-long black flexible scope coiled up in his colon. It was difficult to ascertain whether he was concerned about his condition, cooperating for the sake of getting along, or resigned to his fate.

Two weeks later, his colonoscopy revealed a significant finding—an early rectal cancer, quite superficial at the anorectal junction. One week later he had a surgical resection, and fortunately with early detection he did not require any chemotherapy, radiation or a colostomy. Fifteen years later he remains happy, healthy and cancer-free. I am thankful that I listened to my gut on that first day and avoided a perilous path of least resistance.

A shortsighted medical diagnosis would have been a costly long-term misdiagnosis.

Tim Morrison paid visits to my office generally a few times per year. He was unkempt, with worn-out clothes and suboptimal grooming his trademark. His social history read like a cliched country music song: a messy divorce, difficulty holding down a job, financially strapped, estranged from his two sons. Understandably, he had descended into a deep depression, which had been a challenge to resolve.

A few years ago, he came into my office acutely suicidal, with a plan to run his car into a bridge abutment later that day. That encounter turned into a police visit, followed by transport to the local mental health unit for an involuntary committal for seventy-two hours. It was difficult finding a counselor for him because of his poor insurance coverage, and several of the antidepressant medications that we had tried for him had been ineffective.

After his discharge from the inpatient psychiatric unit, I changed his antidepressant to Zoloft and had him sign a No-Suicide Contract with me while in the office. The substance of this agreement involves the patient making a promise to contact our office, family or police immediately if they become acutely suicidal. Tim signed the contract without reservation, and we arranged for a two-week follow-up visit.

A fortnight later, Tim looked somewhat improved, managing the faint traces of a smile. At last we had found a psychotherapist that accepted his insurance, and finally we found an antidepressant medication which was having some positive impact upon his mood.

I grew cautiously optimistic during our visit. "Well, Tim, things seem to be doing better today. Are you getting into a good place in your life right now?"

Tim's subtle smile flattened ever so slightly, enough for me to notice. "Well Doc, about ten days ago, I finally made up my mind I was gonna do it. Put an end to all of this pain and suffering. I got a sturdy rope, tied one end to the rafter in the garage, the other I shaped into a solid noose. There I was in the garage, rope around my neck, standing on a chair, ready to kick it out from under me and finish the unpleasantness . . ." he trailed off eerily and awkwardly paused. The silence and tension in the room became unbearable. "But then I remembered our contract, and that I promised you that I'd stay safe and not hurt myself. So I couldn't bring myself to do it, I didn't want to let you down. I hope you're not disappointed in my weakest moments."

Holy cow, he had been on the brink of ending it all. "On the contrary, Tim, I'm proud of your courage to fight through life's challenges, to keep showing up every day and trying to do your best. I know that these last few years have been difficult for you and may not get better anytime soon. Please know I'm here for you every step of the way to beat these demons. Just keep me posted on how you're feeling, especially if it's scary depression or suicidal feelings, OK?"

"Sure Doc, you got it. Thanks for having my back." With that, he firmly shook my hand and walked away, his gait a little bit more upright and confident than I had seen previously.

Tim and I have interacted multiple times over the years, and we have tried to keep his depression problem stabilized, despite the recurrent despairing elements of his daily life.

Alice Manning was a delightful ninety-plus-year-old woman who was a patient of one of my clinic partners. She came to see me one early Wednesday morning with some concerns regarding her chronic heart failure. Her weight was up about four pounds, and she was more fatigued and short of breath. Her exam revealed increased fluid-filled crackles about halfway up her lungs, worsening swelling of her legs, and some slight difficulty breathing, even at rest. I reviewed her medication list with her closely and made sure that it was updated and current. Her chest X-ray showed an enlarged heart, increased haziness of the lung fields, and some fluid at the base of the right lung called a pleural effusion.

Her clinical presentation was consistent with a diagnosis of worsening heart failure. Fortunately, she seemed stable enough to go home that day with close observation. I slightly increased the dose of her diuretic to drain more fluid off of her and adjusted her other heart failure medications. She agreed with this approach, and we made a plan to see her back in three days to recheck her clinical progress.

At her follow-up visit, Alice appeared much improved, more comfortable and less anxious. She displayed a noticeable sense of relief at the positive turn of clinical events.

"Thanks Doc, that medication change helped me out a lot. Here, I'd like you to have this." She handed me a gift-wrapped shirt box that was thick and bulging in the middle.

I curiously unwrapped the package and extracted the treasure inside. It was a baby afghan, a panoply of multiple bright blue, pink, and yellow colors, hand-knitted by Alice herself. The multicolored fabric was soft, beautifully elegant and reflected the love and effort invested in creating such a glorious piece of handiwork. It was an overwhelming, wonderful gift, like nothing else that I had ever received.

What happened here a few days ago? All I did was talk to her for a little while, adjusted her medications and that was it. Or was it? All along, was it so much more than diagnoses, medications and test results? At the heart of it all, the coding, documentation and paperwork being thrown at primary care docs like me just isn't that important in the master plan of modern medicine. Maybe there was something more powerful, a primal exchange of emotions, a mutual sense of teamwork to overcome a medical problem, to offer comfort and support, something timeless. My eyes became fluid-filled immediately, and a proud Alice looked lovingly at me and smiled.

"I heard that you have a second baby due any day now, and I thought that you might like to have this blanket. Just finished knitting it recently for no one in particular, guess it was meant for you and your family."

"Wow—this is really precious, I'll treasure it always. Thanks, Alice."

"Thank you, Dr. Rowe, I'll see you around." We hugged each other and she confidently left my office, her newfound mobility and breathability belying her advanced age. Our visit re-centered my focus on the true purpose of serving as a family physician.

With the passage of time, I have developed an understanding of myself and my world to a greater level, and other times to much less of a degree. Confidence and confusion compete like jealous suitors for my time and attention, their objectives increasingly urgent and desperate. Gazing toward an imperfect mirror, my self-image would intermittently deteriorate into unintelligible shadows and smudges of self-doubt before rapidly coalescing again into a brilliant, highly defined picture of life clarity and purpose. I am now fifty years old, and while grateful for my many blessings, my self-confidence occasionally ebbs and flows. I sometimes worry excessively about the what the future holds and my place in it.

It was late August, and I had dropped off my oldest daughter in Iowa City for another year of college at the University of Iowa. *Wow . . . just like Mom and Dad . . . the cycle is repeating itself.* I took a short, spontaneous detour back to my hometown to visit my mom and frequent some of my old haunts in Oskaloosa. All too quickly, it was time to undertake the five-plus-hour trek back to my adopted Wisconsin home. However, there was one more place that was calling to me, some unfinished business to complete.

I drove ten miles farther west to Evergreen Cemetery, out in the middle of the countryside. As I stepped out of my car, the discordant smells of freshly growing corn plants, strong livestock manure and pungent tractor diesel fumes greeted my senses. Though initially jarring to encounter, it was a reassuring reminder of my heritage. I entered the placid graveyard and gazed off into the distance at the green farm fields. The surrounding rows of cornstalks formed a verdant phalanx, tall with burgeoning heavy ears of corn capped with dazzling golden silks. A rolling field of soybeans to the south stretched out in the distance, a rich corduroy Kelly-green carpet. To the west, a confederation of Holstein and Jersey cows lazily grazed in the comfortable, warm afternoon sunlight in a valley by a small creek.

I leisurely walked through the gardens of stone, taking note of the tombstones inscribed with the names of my ancestors: Great-great-grandparents Dries and Janna from Holland, Great-grandparents Neal and Dora, Grandma Helen and Grandpa Herman, and finally Dad, with a sleek black granite tombstone adorned with, what else, a relief of buckeyes. By the fenceposts I found a lantern-like pine cone and a fragrant thick bough of cedar. I knelt down and reverently placed the items at the foot of my father's stone.

As I once again prepared to leave Iowa for an indeterminate period, I contemplated the rows of markers commemorating those who came before me, who risked everything by leaving their old lives in Europe, braving hardships, and losing loved ones too early. The sun was beginning its inevitable late-afternoon trek toward the western horizon, and I poignantly realized that someday my era on earth would mercilessly come to a close. Tomorrow in the east, the sun would return and my descendants would have their chances to make their mark upon the world.

Suddenly, from the northwest a refreshing cool breeze sprung up to greet me. At that moment, I felt the presence of my ancestors in a sense of reassurance. It was a subtle yet perceptible reminder that the days were shortening and the nights were becoming cooler. Though not externally apparent, a change of seasons was rapidly approaching. Soon it would be harvest time, and the rewards for hard work and a job well done would become realized. My extended family tilled these nearby fields for generations, with focused dedication and high hopes for success. The rich topsoil of their work ethic rested upon a solid Midwestern bedrock of clear moral focus, nurtured by a loving blazing sun and cooling rains of kindness. I was inspired to know that they would have similar bold dreams and weighty expectations for the ultimate harvest of my life and my descendant seedlings.

I wistfully started my car and slowly lumbered down the washboarded dusty gravel road back toward the main highway and my hybrid modern reality, warmly basking in the privilege of being a native Iowan. I sincerely hoped that my forefathers would be grateful for the accounting of my life that I strive to improve each and every day and for those around me. Farther down the blacktopped road, as day helplessly gave way to night and the Big Dipper began its steady graceful ascent, I could swear that one of the brighter stars in the constellation was twinkling directly at me.

Probably just a coincidence, but I knew better.

AFTERWORD

One of my objectives in this book was to encourage physicians to explore their own triumphs and setbacks, placing them in proper perspective. All of us are human, and inherently physicians are prone to vulnerabilities and mistakes. I encourage all of you to contemplate the fabric of your lives, and learn from both your positive and negative experiences; but more importantly, embrace the hopefulness and potential of the human condition. As physicians we need to come together in a community of support, celebrating our diversity and skills, and be there for each other when the negative influences of burnout and depression loom large. For those of you who are struggling or going through self-doubt, please reach out to your colleagues and/or a mental health professional—you will be amazed at the support and what others have experienced.

If you have a fascinating patient story that you would like to share with me, I would love to hear from you. Please contact me at my website, listed below, and remember that HIPPA rules apply, so please respect patient privacy. Also, if you enjoyed reading this book, if you could take a couple of minutes to post a positive comment or review on Amazon or the social media platform of your choosing, it would be greatly appreciated.

My contact information is as follows:

Website: bowtiedocblog.com
Twitter: @BruceRoweMD
Instagram: browehawkeye
LinkedIn: linkedin.com/in/bruce-rowe-47391216

ACKNOWLEDGMENTS

A book usually has the names of one or two authors on its cover, but successful writers know they are indebted to an entire community of support that has brought their work to fruition. I am incredibly grateful for my circle of family, coworkers, friends and writing professionals who have been so encouraging in my journey toward writing this book.

Foremost, I would like to thank my family: My wife of twenty-five years, Laura, who has been through many of these joyful and sorrowful experiences with me firsthand, and is my rock; my three daughters, Allison, Chelsea and Julia, who amaze me with their intelligence and moral clarity; my wonderful parents, Sandra and the late Larry Rowe; my incredible in-laws, James and Esther Fus; my special aunt and bibliophile Ernestine Sobczak; my sister Monica Holt, brothers-in-law/sisters-in-law Linda and Robb Guddie, Allison and James Fus, Jr., for the gift of their love and friendship and creating such special memories together.

My colleagues and coworkers at the Glendale Clinic/Ascension Medical Group in Brown Deer have been critical to my personal growth and in the success of our physicians' medical practices. I especially would like to thank my medical assistant of nearly fifteen years, Latisha Ward; my lead triage nurse, Jodie Falk; our wonderful nurses, medical assistants and nurse practitioners; my fellow family physicians: Drs. Francisca Olmedo-Estrada, Gregory Matthews, Michael Plotkin, Robert Kitsis, Michael Johnstone, Michael Fetherston, David Hadcock, Lisa Speidel and Heather Ho, as well as the multiple specialists that work in our office and support us every day. I also appreciate the unique guidance and inspiration from my former colleagues in family practice: Drs. Joseph Schwind, Curtis Kommer and the late Michael Richter. I am grateful for the daily support from our tremendous front desk reception, lab, radiology and therapy departments. Thanks to my Clinic Operations Manager, Angie Dienhart, and my Regional Director, Patti Paulus, for their hard work behind the scenes to make our clinic successful. Emile Dalal, our long-serving pharmacist in our clinic, was always a unique character. To Drs. William DiGilio, Robert Roth, Drew Elgin, Kenneth Johnson, Barry Gimbel, Domenic Pulito, Fred Westreich, and Stephen Sievers, thanks for being such great role models and showing me what it truly means to be a great physician.

To my special friends in the Mequon community, thank you for making our lives joyful and rewarding through the gifts of love and support. For inspiration toward generating this book, I especially appreciate the encouragement of my friends Jim and Lauren Schrier, Jeff and Theresa Phelps, as well as Robert and Polly Schellinger.

For the guidance with the writing process, I am grateful for the insights of my editor, Stuart Horwitz of Book Architecture, and my informal literary consultants, Lisa Tener and Jill Grimes. Thanks to the team at 1106 Design, including Michele DeFilippo, Ronda Rawlins, Brian Smith and other staff that worked on my project, for all of their insights and expertise, and for teaching me the intricacies of the book publishing journey.

To my dear patients, thank you for allowing me to share your stories with the world, and for educating and enriching me with your inspiring medical tales. Finally, I thank you, kind reader, for allowing me to come into your lives and share this deeply personal story with you. I hope that you enjoyed reading this book as much as my labor of love in its creation.

ABOUT THE AUTHOR

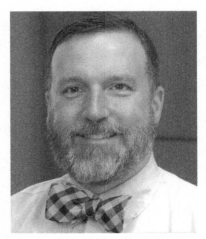

A native of Oskaloosa, a small county seat in southeastern Iowa, Dr. Rowe earned his Doctor of Medicine degree from The University of Iowa and completed residency training in family medicine at the Medical College of Wisconsin-Waukesha. For the last two-plus decades, he has been an attending physician at the Ascension-Columbia St. Mary's Clinic in Brown Deer, Wisconsin. He enjoys the complexity and variety of primary care medicine, but most importantly, the joyful opportunity to enter into deeply personal therapeutic relationships with individuals from all walks of life. He lives in suburban Milwaukee, Wisconsin with his wife Laura, three daughters and a playful cockapoo named Sasha.

Made in the USA
Coppell, TX
28 May 2020